Dictionary of
Psychiatry

Edited by

HENRY WALTON
MD, PhD, FRCPE, FRCPsych
Professor of Psychiatry
University of Edinburgh

BLACKWELL
SCIENTIFIC PUBLICATIONS
OXFORD LONDON EDINBURGH
BOSTON PALO ALTO MELBOURNE

© 1985 by
Blackwell Scientific Publications
Editorial offices:
Osney Mead, Oxford, OX2 0EL
8 John Street, London, WC1N 2ES
23 Ainslie Place, Edinburgh,
  EH3 6AJ
52 Beacon Street, Boston
  Massachusetts 02108, USA
667 Lytton Avenue, Palo Alto
  California 94301, USA
107 Barry Street, Carlton
  Victoria 3053, Australia

First published 1985

Printed in Great Britain by
The Alden Press, Oxford

DISTRIBUTORS

USA
  Blackwell Mosby Book
    Distributors
  11830 Westline Industrial Drive
  St Louis, Missouri 63141

Canada
  Blackwell Mosby Book
    Distributors
  120 Melford Drive, Scarborough
  Ontario M1B 2X4

Australia
  Blackwell Scientific Publications
    (Australia) Pty Ltd
  107 Barry Street
  Carlton, Victoria 3053

British Library
Cataloguing in Publication Data

Dictionary of psychiatry.
  1. Psychiatry—Dictionaries
  I. Walton, Henry J.
  616.89'003'21   RC437

  ISBN 0–632–00972–1

Contributors

J.H.J. BANCROFT MD FRCPsych DPM, *Honorary Senior Lecturer, Department of Psychiatry, University of Edinburgh*

S. BRANDON MD DCH MRCP FRCPsych DPM, *Professor of Psychiatry, University of Leicester*

R.H. CAWLEY PhD FRCP FRCPsych, *Professor of Psychiatry, King's College Hospital Medical School and Institute of Psychiatry, University of London*

F.A. JENNER PhD FRCP FRCPsych DPM, *Professor of Psychiatry, University of Sheffield*

J.B. LOUDON MB ChB FRCPsych DPM, *Consultant Psychiatrist, Royal Edinburgh Hospital*

S. MALITZ MD, FRCPsych, *Professor of Psychiatry, College of Physicians and Surgeons of Columbia University, New York*

Sir DESMOND POND MD FRCP FRCPsych DPM, *Chief Scientist, Department of Health and Social Security, Past President, Royal College of Psychiatrists, formerly Professor of Psychiatry, London Hospital Medical College, University of London*

V. RAKOFF MB BS FRCP(C), *Professor and Chairman, Department of Psychiatry and Clarke Institute of Psychiatry, University of Toronto*

K. RAWNSLEY CBE FRCPsych FRCP DPM, *President, Royal College of Psychiatrists, Professor of Psychological Medicine, University of Wales College of Medicine, Cardiff*

Sir MARTIN ROTH MD FRCP FRCPsych DPM, *Professor of Psychiatry, University of Cambridge*

G.E. RUFF MD, *Professor of Psychiatry, University of Pennsylvania, Philadelphia*

Contributors

R.L. SPITZER MD, *Chief of Psychiatric Research, Biometrics Research Department, New York State Psychiatric Institute, New York*

H.J. WALTON MD PhD FRCPE FRCPsych MD(Hon)Uppsala DPM, *Professor of Psychiatry, University of Edinburgh, Consultant Psychiatrist, Royal Edinburgh Hospital and Western General Hospital, Edinburgh. President, World Federation for Medical Education*

Foreword

The student, entering the world of psychiatry and the behavioural sciences, encounters a vocabulary which is at once strange and familiar. Words such as 'depression' or 'hysteria', common in lay parlance, may have a very different meaning technically. Further confusion is generated by the discovery that even within the scientific and professional body, many terms, e.g. schizophrenia or psychopath, enjoy a variety of meanings when used by different authorities.

Recognition of this difficulty prompted the World Health Organization to publish a glossary of diagnostic terms in conjunction with the Mental Disorders Section of the *International Classification of Diseases* 9th Revision – a remarkable achievement of apparent harmony in a contentious field.

The present dictionary embodies a response to the expressed need for an authoritative, accessible and compact set of definitions and explanations of words used in psychiatry and cognate subjects.

It has been compiled by a panel of British and American psychiatrists and provides an invaluable source of information for psychiatrists, both established and in training, and for other doctors. The work will appeal to a wider readership within the health professions: nurses, psychologists, social workers, administrators and to many groups outside, lawyers, magistrates, journalists and interested members of the public.

1985   K. Rawnsley
                                  President
                                  Royal College of Psychiatrists

abreaction   The expression or discharge of strong **emotion**, previously concealed or repressed, occurring spontaneously or as a reaction to a stirring experience, or in response to verbal exchanges during the course of **psychotherapy**. It may be deliberately provoked by **drugs**, either as an investigative procedure or for therapeutic purposes.

abstinence syndrome   *See* **Withdrawal syndrome.**

accommodation   *See* **Piaget.**

acromegaly   Clinical manifestation of pituitary tumour producing excess of growth hormone in adults. Clinical features include changes in facial features and overgrowth of the head, hands and feet. Headaches and visual disturbances occur due to mechanical effects of the tumour. Most common psychological **symptoms** are emotional instability, apathy, impairment of sexual function, lack of initiative and disturbance of recent memory.

acting out   A term often applied to the occurrence of unreasonable **behaviour** as partial expression of emotional tension. Originally it described the **displacement** of a behavioural response from one situation to another during the course of **psychotherapy**. Usually this involves **transference**, with the projection of feelings towards the therapist on to others in the environment, e.g. a child or a spouse.

adaptation   Change in **behaviour** that fits the person more adequately for the environmental conditions, e.g. a modification in impulses, **emotions** or attitudes.

addict   A person who develops **addiction**. In current usage, physiological and psychological **dependence** on the substance are stressed.

addiction   **Dependence physical** or **psychological** on chemical substances (e.g. drugs, **alcohol**) leading to a **compulsion** to take the substance continuously to experience its effects, and sometimes to avoid the discomfort of its absence. **Tolerance** may occur, increasing the amount of the substance needed to bring about the same effect.

adjustment   Successful **adaptation**; achievement by the individual of equilibrium between himself and his external environment, or between himself and his inner psychological environment, so that unconscious **conflicts** are coped with.

Adler, Alfred (1870–1937)   Early associate of **Freud** who later developed his own school of **individual psychology**. Believed the struggle for power, self-respect and recognition was of central importance with the associated development of an inferiority **complex** because of one's apparent failures. He also emphasized **overcompensation** as a mechanism to deal with perceived defects of the self, e.g. the partially deaf's love of music.

adolescence Developmental stage beginning with the onset of **puberty** (age 11–13) and ending with the achievement of young adulthood. It is characterized by physical and emotional maturation, psychological **adaptation** and full sexual development. The many changes occurring during this period and the rapidity and complexity of their interaction frequently result in periods of **stress** in an attempt to cope successfully with these alterations. *See also* **behaviour**.

aerophagy Excessive air swallowing, sometimes associated with noisy eructations and sometimes with abdominal distension.

aetiology Causative factors in illness. These include specific factors if known (such as bacteria), **genetic** vulnerability, constitutional predisposition and environmental influences.
precipitating aetiology Factors which can be inherited, acquired or which are in the environment, and operate to start off an illness or disorder, to which the patient may have been constitutionally liable.

affect Feeling, **emotion** or **mood**; the feeling accompanying a particular idea.
incongruity of affect An emotional response which is not in keeping with the content of the patient's **thoughts**, or with the circumstances in which he finds himself and the experiences that elicit them.
poverty of affect A substantial narrowing of the range of emotional response to situations, with blunting or inadequacy of **mood**; can extend to a loss of emotional life.

affective disorder Disorder in which **mood** change is the main abnormality, from which other **symptoms** are derived. Chief are depressive and manic **psychosis**, but **anxiety** states are also included in most classifications. Recovery from an episode of affective illness is usually complete, no matter how frequent recurrence is. *See also* **depressive illness**.

bipolar affective disorder Affective illness showing episodes both of **depressive illness** and of **mania** or **hypomania**.

postpartum affective disorder Although **mania** is not common after childbirth, mixed mood disorders are, and with acute onset and **clouding** of **consciousness** they may closely resemble

schizophrenia. They do however carry a much better prognosis, though approximately 1 in 3 will experience a recurrence in a subsequent pregnancy. In both depressive and mixed states there is a risk of **infanticide**. *See also* **depressive illness, postpartum; psychosis, puerperal.**

unipolar affective disorder An affective disorder in which the patient's condition (usually in the form of episodes or attacks) manifests itself in only one clinical form, e.g. recurrent **depressive illness** without **manic** episodes in addition.

after image On looking away from a bright light a series of similar positive images (of the same quality as the light) and negative images (its opposite quality) persist for many seconds. Such after images are partly from the eye (retinal) and partly of brain origin. Comparable after effects occur with other sensory inputs (e.g. motion, posture). After images are of universal distribution and of no known special psychological significance.

aggression A forceful physical or verbal action, accompanied by the **affect** of anger, rage or hostility. It may be as realistic and adaptive as self-assertiveness, or morbid when unrealistic, self-destructive, inappropriately harmful to others, and an expression of unresolved emotional **conflicts**.

agitation Marked tension and restlessness associated with severe **anxiety** or depressed **mood**. In severe cases the patient may be unable to be still or concentrate for more than a few seconds, and the **thought** content is scattered but anxiety-laden. Occasionally **senile** patients may give the impression of agitation through their constant restlessness.

agnosia A disorder of the parietal lobes of the brain whereby the patient cannot interpret sensations correctly, although the sense organs and the nerves conducting sensation to the brain are functioning normally. In visual agnosia the patient can see but cannot recognize objects, including letters. In auditory agnosia the patient can hear but cannot interpret speech or other sounds. In tactile agnosia the patient has normal sensation in his hands but cannot identify objects by touch alone.

agoraphobia Specific fear of being alone, or being away from home or of being in public places. The individual avoids crowds or other situations in which panic and physical **symptoms** of **anxiety** may occur.

agraphia An acquired inability to write either spontaneously or to dictation, although there is no weakness or inco-ordination of the hand. Results from disease in or damage to the parietal lobe of the brain, and is related to the disorders of language (**aphasia**). Also occurs in association with **dyspraxia**.

Agrippa, Cornelius (ca. 1486–1535) Wandering scholar who in 1519 risked his life at Metz to free a woman accused of witchcraft. An early critic of the demonological notion of insanity, he influenced **Weyer** to reject the belief in witchcraft and to study those stigmatized as witches by clinical observation and examination.

akathisia (lit. inability to sit) An old term applied to the paradoxical restlessness seen in otherwise relatively immobile **Parkinsonism**, now revived to apply to similar fidgetiness often present in some patients taking **tranquillizers**, especially **phenothiazines**. The patient may complain of inner tension as well as exhibit limb and facial movements of voluntary type.

akinesis (lit. absence of movement) Most commonly seen in adjectival form, the exact meaning then depending on the state thus qualified, e.g. akinetic **catatonia**, akinetic **mutism**, akinetic **epileptic seizures**. *See also* **dyskinesis**.

alcohol abuse Drinking alcohol in a manner which causes harm to oneself or others.

alcohol dependence (syn. alcohol **addiction**, alcoholism) The syndrome consisting of psychological and physical **symptoms** including increasing use of alcohol in daily life, subjective feelings of needing a drink, **withdrawal symptoms** (i.e. **anxiety, tremor**, restlessness) and drinking to relieve withdrawal symptoms; **delirium tremens** a severe form. Chronic severe addiction leads to disorder of the heart muscle, peripheral neuritis, cirrhosis of the liver and brain impairment.

alcohol intoxication **Symptoms** from excessive intake, consisting of unsteadiness of the limbs and gait, slurring of speech, impairment of the intellectual functions and loss of **inhibitions**, often terminating in **sleep**.

alcoholic A term for one who is addicted to alcohol and has adverse consequences from drinking, including impairment of physical or mental health, disturbance of personal relationships, and impaired performance at work. *See also* **hallucinosis**.

Alcoholics Anonymous An international voluntary self-help agency for **alcoholics**, organized and operated locally. The members are regarded as having an illness, but must accept responsibility to become abstinent, while openly discussing drink problems in the past and current difficulties with sobriety at regular meetings; members undertake to help other members, promoting friendship and altruism.

alcoholism A state of **addiction** to alcohol, when psychological or physical **dependence**, or both, have developed. One of the most serious of contemporary public health problems because of its prevalence and the manifold types of alcohol-related harm resulting to the **alcoholic** and others with whom he is associated.

Alexander, Franz (1891–1964) Psychoanalyst who, when in Chicago, developed theories associating specific **psychosomatic illnesses** with typical **conflicts**, a view now rarely accepted.

Alzheimer's disease A progressive form of **dementia** due to diffuse degeneration of the brain and occurring in middle age. Commences with **memory** impairment associated with **mood** disturbance, incompetence in ordinary tasks and **disorientation** for space. Focal symptoms follow from lesions in the parietal lobes: disorganization of speech, **apraxia, agnosia** and difficulty with calculation. In recent years a unitary concept of Alzheimer's disease has gained wide acceptance. In consequence, the terms Senile Dementia of Alzheimer's Type (SDAT) and Pre-senile Dementia of Alzheimer's Type (PDAT) are commonly used. Although it is recognised that the two syndromes are separated by some distinctive clinical features, it is considered that they are varying manifestations of a unitary aetiological process and that the nomenclature should reflect this. *See also* **dementia senile, dementia simple** and **dementia presenile**.

ambivalence Coexistence of opposed and contradictory **emotions** (such as love and hate), attitudes or impulses related to a person or situation. May be expressed in **behaviour** or utterances, leading to indecisiveness or **obsessions**, which may be accompanied by conscious awareness of the contradiction. In **psychodynamic psychiatry** ambivalence is held to derive from emotional **conflict**.

amenorrhoea The absence of menstruation which may be primary, when menses have never appeared, or secondary when there is interruption of a previously established menstrual rhythm. *See* **anorexia nervosa.**

amines   *See* **brain amines**.

amnesia   Loss of **memory** following brain disease or injury, **drugs** or psychological causes.

posthypnotic amnesia   An island of **memory** impairment deliberately induced in a hypnotized subject. Refers to an inability to recall or sometimes to recognize certain items or areas of experience which can subsequently be regained either by further **suggestion** by the hypnotist or spontaneously.

post-traumatic amnesia   The **memory** loss following an injury, most often to the brain, which extends backward to affect experience prior to the injury (retrograde) and sometimes that subsequent to it (anterograde).

retrograde amnesia   The **memory** loss due to a (usually closed) head injury that prevents recollection of events immediately preceding the trauma. The length of the gap is a good measure of the severity of the injury. It is caused mainly by a failure of registration but vague fleeting memories can sometimes be recalled subsequently.

amnesic syndrome   An organic brain impairment in which the predominant disturbance is profound **memory** loss, mainly for recent events. An example of the amnesic syndrome is **Korsakoff psychosis**.

amok   Occurs in South-East Asia and parts of Africa. After withdrawal and brooking commonly, the person runs wild, attacking and often killing a series of victims indiscriminately; before collapsing or being overpowered.

amphetamine   A **stimulant drug** which increases wakefulness, concentration and energy, decreases fatigue and suppresses appetite. The aftermath of amphetamine use is characterized by a reversal of these effects. It acts by releasing catecholamines from presynaptic storage sites in the brain.

amphetamine abuse   Non-medical use of many forms. May be as an aid to slimming, occasional use to elevate **mood**, or true **addiction** when **sedatives** may be taken in addition. Chronic excessive use can lead to development of a toxic **psychosis**, indistinguishable from **paranoid schizophrenia**, which usually disappears when the **drug** is stopped.

amphetamine addiction   **Dependence** on amphetamine, a serious complication usually of non-medical use. *See also* **amphetamine abuse**.

amphetamine psychosis   Organic mental illness due to the drug, most often characterized by **paranoid delusions**.

anaclitic   (lit. leaning on) Refers to relationships which are characterized by **dependence** on others, e.g. the position the infant is in with its mother. Anaclitic depression, which may manifest as failure to thrive, may occur with sudden separation of the infant from the mother. In **psychotherapy**, planned gratification of a patient's dependency needs, in a closely supportive relationship with the clinician.

anal stage   The second **pregenital** stage of **personality development** in **psychoanalytic theory**, associated with sensuous pleasure related to defaecation or retention of faeces, and forming the centre of the infant's self-awareness. Often referred to as the anal-sadistic stage and related to mastery of the body, especially the sphincters, when socialization of impulses is the infant's major preoccupation; and in adulthood to certain regressive **personality** traits and to obsessional symptoms. *See* **obsession.**

analgesics   Pain-relieving **drugs**, including the **opiates,** whose action is at specific **receptor** sites in the brain, and anti-inflammatory drugs such as aspirin whose site of action is local.

analysand   A person or patient undergoing **psychoanalysis.**

analysis   *See* **psychoanalysis**.

analytical psychology   *See* **Jung.**

anamnesis   An old term, now little used, referring to recollections by the patient when the medical history is obtained.

anankastic personality disorder   *See* **personality disorder, obsessional**.

anankastic symptoms   *See* **neurosis, obsessional**.

anhedonia   The absence of pleasure in acts or experiences which are normally pleasurable. Occurs, for example, in the **borderline state** and in **schizophrenia**.

animal magnetism   Historical term due to **Mesmer,** who worked in Vienna and Paris and postulated that a magnetic fluid fills the universe and continually flows within and around every human being, whose state of health is determined by the harmonious balance

animism

of the fluid. Mesmer claimed that he could magnetize a sick person, and thus alter the flow in or out, to restore health. Now obsolete, his ideas provided the basis for later discoveries of **hypnosis** and **suggestion**.

animism   The second stage of intellectual development, between the ages of 2 and 7 years, for which **Piaget** has described four principal characteristics: egocentrism, animism, preoperational logic and an authoritarian morality. Animism implies that everything is alive and has feelings and thoughts, every event occurs by intent, eg. the wind blows because it wants to; the table against which the child bumps his head is 'naughty'.

animus   *See* **Jung.**

anomie   (lit. without law) A lack of connection and identification with the laws and customs of a society. Often used to convey social marginality and alienation. In many instances thought to be a consequence of abrupt social and economic transitions and the dissolution of supportive social contexts. Identified by **Durkheim** as a major cause of **suicide**.

anorexia   Lack or loss of appetite.

anorexia nervosa   A well-recognized psychiatric **syndrome** first described by Sir William Gull (1816-1890) and consisting of a persistent active refusal to eat, marked loss of weight and persistent **amenorrhoea**. Characteristically, the disorder begins in teenage girls but it may occur before **puberty.** Rarely occurs in boys. There is often a remarkably high level of alertness and physical activity even when the stage of gross emaciation is reached. Many cases show a characteristic weight **phobia**, a continuous preoccupation with food, a **body image disorder**, and unusual eating habits or attitudes to food including stealing or hoarding food and alternate periods of starvation or overeating sometimes associated with vomiting or purgation.

antabuse   *See* **disulfiram.**

anticonvulsants   **Drugs** which given in doses that do not produce unacceptable drowsiness or other undesirable side-effects completely or partially suppress **fits (convulsions)** in **epilepsy** of various types.

antidepressant drugs   Compounds used to treat the **symptoms** found in major **depressive illness**, including abnormalities of **mood**, sleeping, thinking and **sexual** functioning. Their main action is on cerebral monoamines and associated **receptors**, and the effect occurs only after a number of days. The most commonly used are **tricyclic antidepressant drugs** and the **monoamine oxidase inhibitors.**

anti-Parkinsonism drugs Drugs with anticholinergic effects in the **central nervous system** that can be used to provide symptomatic relief in **Parkinsonism** or the drug-induced **extrapyramidal** syndromes.

antisocial 1. Opposed to the interests or rules of society. 2. (sl.) Shunning social contact. *See also* **personality disorder, sociopathic**.

anxiety A state of uneasy concern in response to external events or inner **thoughts** and feelings or, in **psychoanalytic theory**, due to conflict associated with **unconscious** repressed impulses. It may be experienced as an unpleasant **emotion**, with elements of **fear** and dread. It may be expressed verbally, or in other **behaviour**, and in a characteristic state of physiological arousal. The experience and expression of anxiety are normal when appropriate to and focused on particular situations. When they are free-floating, pervasive and excessive, they reflect an abnormal or pathological state.

anxiety disorder *See* **neurosis, anxiety**.

anxiety symptoms **Symptoms** attributable to **anxiety**, including psychological symptoms such as tension, feelings of apprehension and dread, restlessness, inappropriate **fear**; and physical symptoms including palpitations, sweating, trembling, and other manifestations of **autonomic nervous system** arousal.

anxiolytic drugs Medication with anti-**anxiety** effect, very widely prescribed to relieve emotional tension. Often referred to as minor **tranquillizers**. Commonly used are the **benzodiazepines; barbiturates** are now much less used because they are addictive and have unhelpful **sedative** effects in addition.

apathy Relative lack of feeling; a state of the **emotions** in which responsiveness is reduced or lacking.

aphasia Loss, either partial or complete, of the ability to express oneself verbally or to comprehend the meaning of language, resulting from damage to the speech area of the brain. Stroke is the most common cause. Nominal aphasia is inability to express the right word.

aphonia

aphonia   Inability to produce sound when mouthing words. A common type is based on psychological **conflicts** and has been called **hysterical**. May respond to intravenous **benzodiazepine** and **suggestion**. May also be caused by severe throat inflammation, infection or diseases of the larynx. In such cases the patient is unable to cough, whereas in functional cases the ability to cough audibly is retained. **hysterical aphonia**   Loss of voice, without physical cause, which is believed to result from **unconscious** psychological **conflict**.

apraxia   *See* **dyspraxia**.

arson   Pathological impulse to cause fires. Syn. incendiarism. *See also* **pyromania**.

arteriosclerosis, cerebral   *See* **cerebral arteriosclerosis**.

arteriosclerotic dementia   *See* **dementia**.

Asperger, Hans   German paediatrician. *See* **Asperger's syndrome**.

Asperger's Syndrome   A condition of middle childhood described by Asperger in 1944 consisting of enduring personality traits of solitariness, constricted interests, unusual modes of thinking, heightened sensitivity and lack of empathy, sometimes accompanied by general or specific developmental retardation, and thought to have a genetic basis. It is much commoner in boys. There are similarities with **early infantile autism**, and it has been linked to **schizoid personality disorder** in adult life.

assimilation   *See* **Piaget**.

associationism   The dominant school of **psychology** of the mid-nineteenth century, in which it was postulated that all psychological data can be broken down into simple elements (sensations or ideas), and that most if not all human experience and **behaviour** can be explained in terms of the **complexes** formed according to the laws of association, by the coming together in space and time, or by similarity in content, of groups of these elements.

astasia-abasia   A form of **hysterical** unsteadiness of gait (ataxia) characterized by bizarre inco-ordination and inability to walk or stand even though all leg movements can be performed normally while sitting or lying down.

asthenic type   One of **Kretschmer's** constitutional types, of individuals who are lean in **physique** and cold and detached in **personality**.

asthma   Paroxysmal attacks of difficulty in breathing with wheezing cough and a sense of constriction, due to spasm of the bronchi. Attacks may be precipitated by a large range of stimuli, includings allergens and emotional **stress**, in a physiologically susceptible person. A number of **psychogenic** factors have been cited, in particular actual or fantasied separation from the protective mother, but any form of psychic stress may generate an attack in a vulnerable individual.

asylum   A refuge or sanctuary for the shelter and protection of individuals otherwise at risk. The term mental (or **lunatic**) asylum was once used for institutions for the treatment and care of the mentally ill.

ataractic   The effect of tranquillizers in diminishing **anxiety** and producing a state of calmness. *See also* **neuroleptics**.

athletic type   *See* **physique**.

attachment   The propensity of human beings to make strong emotional bonds to other people significant to them. Interference with attachment can give rise to many forms of emotional distress, including **anxiety**, anger, depression and emotional detachment. In mammals the first and most persistent **bonding** is between mother and young.

attention   The selective focusing of the conscious mental activity of the moment on certain objects or **thoughts**, to the relative exclusion of others.

short attention span   (syn. **distractibility**) Inability to sustain focused mental activity on particular objects or **thoughts** for an appropriate period of time.

auditory agnosia   *See* **agnosia**.

aura   A brief sensory experience (lasting seconds) preceding an attack, which in the current usage of the word is epileptic in nature, but in the past could apply to any subsequent disturbance of **consciousness**.
epileptic aura   Brief motor, sensory, **autonomic** or psychological **symptoms** marking the onset of an epileptic attack. The nature of the symptoms depends on the brain area in which the attack begins. Epileptic auras are of great variety, the commonest being those

autism

occurring in temporal lobe **epilepsy**. Epileptic auras are regarded as being the result of a focal epileptic discharge, thus distinguishing them from epileptic **prodrome**. *See also* **epilepsy**.

autism   A condition of withdrawing from realistic **attention** to the environment, to a state of thinking determined solely by wishes and **fantasies** unrelated to external reality; a **symptom** of disorder such as **schizophrenia**, or of **personality disorder**. *See also* **early infantile autism**.

autistic   Mental activity that is predominantly subjective and detached from reality. *See also* **autism**.

autistic thought   *See* **thought**.

auto-erotism   Sexual stimulation not involving active participation of a partner, e.g. erotic **fantasy** or **masturbation**.

automatic obedience   Uncritical response to commands often in a setting of hypersuggestibility, sometimes found in **schizophrenia**.

automatic writing   A feature of certain dissociative states in which the subject writes material which discloses **thoughts** or feelings of which he is unaware. **Consciousness** may be altered, with the individual in a **trance**-like state, or normal, in which case the **automatism** is confined to the movements of the arm and hand.

automatism   A sequence of actions performed without conscious thought, usually applied to a pathological **dissociation** of **consciousness** and **behaviour** resulting from **epilepsy, hysterical** illness or other causes. However, it can be applied to normal complex acts carried out without conscious control. The acts may be simple and repetitive or complex and apparently goal-seeking.

autonomic nervous system   The part of the nervous system responsible for the control of physical functions that are not consciously directed, e.g. breathing, the heart beat, intestinal movements, sweating etc. Subdivided into two systems: the sympathetic nerve endings release noradrenaline and the parasympathetic acetylcholine. Sympathetic effects on organs may be excitatory such as contraction of the bowel sphincters, constriction of the blood vessels and increase in heart rate. Sympathetic overactivity occurs in certain psychiatric illnesses, e.g. agitated depressive **psychosis**, acute **schizophrenia** and anxiety **neurosis**.

autoscopy   (lit. viewing of self) In practice applied usually only to brief abnormal **perceptions** or **hallucinations** of parts of the body, even of inside organs, that can occur as an epileptic **aura** or more rarely in **schizophrenia**.

autosuggestibility   Heightened receptiveness to ideas from within; undue tendency to accept and act upon notions the person has himself, elaborated either consciously or unconsciously.

aversion therapy   Psychological treatment approach by which the stimulus towards undesired **behaviour** (e.g. craving for alcohol) is associated with an aversive stimulus (e.g. induction of vomiting by the drug apomorphine, or electric shock) with the aim of inhibiting the behaviour.

Babinski, Joseph (1857–1932)   Follower of **Charcot** who refined the concept of hysteria to that which could be produced by or suppressed by **suggestion**. He is particularly famous for introducing the toe sign or Babinski sign to differentiate organic from hysterical states: in leg weakness of physical cause (upper motor neurone lesions) the big toe is extended when the outer edge of the sole is scraped; normally the big toe flexes.

barbiturate addiction   A **syndrome** of physical and psychological **dependence** similar in many respects to chronic **alcoholism**. Chronic **intoxication** is associated with gross deterioration of **personality** and marked signs of brain toxicity. The **withdrawal** (or abstinence) **syndrome** appears after 12-16 hours and consists of **anxiety,** tachycardia, weakness, tremulousness, muscle fasciculation, **anorexia**, vomiting, abdominal distress, increased startle response and in many **addicts, convulsions** or **psychosis**.

barbiturates   A group of **drugs** derived from barbituric acid, with **depressant** effects on the brain ranging from sedation to **coma**. They have been used as hypnotic, anaesthetic and antiepileptic agents. Because they may easily produce **physical** and **psychological dependence** they are now rarely used as **hypnotics**.

Bateson, Gregory (1904–1980)   Biologist and anthropologist interested also in **psychiatry**. He introduced the concept of the **doublebind**, erroneously postulated as causal in **schizophrenia**. For example, the child is given contradictory messages simultaneously by a parent (loving intentions may be conveyed in an angry tone of voice) and cannot possibly respond properly.

battered baby syndrome *See* **non-accidental injury**.

battle fatigue The grossly incapacitating responses of soldiers to the dangers of combat. These can be dazed states, profound **anxiety** reactions, **depression, hallucinatory states**, or complete shock and exhaustion.

Beers, Clifford W. (1876–1943) His book about his psychiatric illness, *A Mind That Found Itself* (1909) was followed by the founding of the National Committee for Mental Hygiene in New York, with which he was assisted by **Adolf Meyer** and **William James**.

behaviour The total response which a person makes in any situation. The observable activity of an organism is the definition adopted by behaviourists, but most students of mental processes include experience available to **introspection**, such as ideas, **thoughts**, images **dreams, obsessions** etc.

adolescent behaviour problems Disturbances in behaviour occurring during **adolescence** and associated with or attributed to the individual's emotional growth, which is rapid but as yet incomplete. Behaviour is unstable and subject to **conflict** with external reality and control, particularly by persons in authority.

antisocial behaviour Generally hostile, unfriendly, antagonistic behaviour, often including attitudes of indifference to social mores and rules, as well as violation of conventional property rights and status hierarchies. Includes misbehaviour, **pathological lying**, stealing, physical violence and **sexual deviation.** Common in **childhood behaviour disorders** and sociopathic **personality disorder**, but not necessarily indicative of mental disorder.

childhood behaviour disorders A term for disturbances of behaviour and emotion seen in children. Includes antisocial conduct such as aggressiveness, disobedience, stealing, **truancy**, running away from home, and fire-setting; and also disturbances of emotion (or **neurotic** disorders) including **anxiety**, fears, **depression** and relationship difficulties.

behaviour modification The clinical application of psychological learning principles in order to help a patient change his behaviour. *See also* **behaviour therapy**.

behaviour therapy Treatment of psychological disturbance through an approach directed at unlearning faulty or limiting behaviour or responses e.g. **phobias**. The therapy is directed at the problem behaviour (*See* **desensitization, aversion therapy**) and not at a defined illness process or presumed unconscious **conflict**.

behaviourism An approach in **psychology** holding that only observable **behaviour** need be studied, thus dispensing with attempts to grasp what the patient's experiences are like (*See* **empathy**), and denying that **unconscious** processes have relevance.

beliefs **Thoughts**, ideas and concepts, moulded by education, religion and parental influence, which play a major role in opinion and **behaviour**.

collective beliefs Usually refers to concepts of smaller subcultural groups, but also in **analytical psychology** to widespread innate ideas of a so-called shared collective **mind**.

false beliefs Ideas which are patently untrue. When shared by a group, **superstitions**; when singular in a psychiatrically ill person, **delusions**.

belle indifférence A bland indifference to distressing **symptoms** in **hysterical** illness, the latter due to **conversion** of internal emotional **conflicts** which leads to some resolution of the patient's current personal problems.

benzodiazepines The generic name for a series of compounds which have come to be extremely commonly prescribed, with excellent safety margin and low abuse potential. They are used for the symptomatic relief of **anxiety** and **insomnia**. **Chlordiazepoxide** is the prototype **drug**.

bereavement The loss of a loved person, usually a relative or close friend. **Mourning** or normal **grief** is the response to bereavement and enables the individual to come to terms with the loss.

bestiality Sexual contact with an animal, taking the form of anal or vaginal intercourse, **fellatio** or **masturbation**.

Binet, Alfred (1857–1911) French psychologist who with Theodore Simon in 1905 introduced **intelligence tests**. The Stanford-Binet tests are an American revision of 1916.

binge Heavy continuous drinking leading to sustained high blood alcohol; may last an evening or a month, but has a beginning and an end. Also used to describe to periodic excessive food intake.

Binswanger, Ludwig (1881–1966) Swiss psychiatrist who introduced *Daseinanalyse* as a treatment method in **psychiatry**. This is based on the philosophical works of **Heidegger** and **Husserl**. **Schizophrenia**, for example, was to be seen differently from the traditional conceptual approach of psychiatry and the patient given

biofeedback

an authentically human outlook on the world through an existential psychotherapeutic approach. *See also* **psychiatry, existential**.

biofeedback   Those techniques used to increase subjective awareness of bodily functions, especially muscle tension, blood pressure and heart rate, by their instrumental measurement and display as sound, light or meter readings. This allows one to learn self-control of such functions, in fact usually to relax. Has been used to treat **anxiety, migraine**, hypertension, headaches etc.

bipolar disorder   *See* **affective disorder; depressive illness; psychosis, manic-depressive.**

birth trauma   Obsolete concept, originally proposed by Otto Rank, that the process of birth is a traumatic experience which is remembered in some form, its **recall** or re-enactment being a factor in the later development of **anxiety.**

blackouts   A non-specific term covering attacks in which **consciousness** is temporarily suspended or altered in some way. Used often by **alcoholics** to describe difficulty in recalling events during drinking.

Bleuler, Eugene (1857–1939)   Swiss psychiatrist who coined the term **schizophrenia**, for a group of illnesses in which **dissociation** of ideas, **autism**, loss of **rapport**, **incongruity of affect** and poverty of ideas are basic **symptoms**, and **delusions, hallucinations**, loss of **memory**, disintegration of the **personality** etc. are secondary developments. Much of Bleuler's work is a bringing together of the views of **Freud** and **Kraepelin**.

body image disorder   Disturbance of the internal representation a person has of the body, its size, shape and integral nature. Occurs in brain disease, especially when the parietal lobes are affected, and in psychiatric illness.

bondage   Sexual pleasure in relation to humiliation, physical restriction of movement or danger. *See also* **masochism**.

bonding   Development of **attachment** between persons in a relationship, e.g. a mother and her baby. *See also* **emotional bonding**.

borderline state   Refers to those patients who are not obviously **psychotic** but on the verge of, or capable of, decompensating into frank psychotic illness. In recent years used to describe a **personality** state characterized by impulsive **acting-out** behaviour, disturbances of **mood** and interpersonal relationships, and self destructive acts, with **identity** disturbance as the core impairment. *See also* **schizophrenia, latent and pseudoneurotic**.

bout drinker (Syn. episodic or periodic drinker). A person who spaces out heavy drinking by periods of relative or complete abstinence lasting three or more days, or often several weeks. May move from being a continuous drinker to being a bout drinker, and change back again, depending on lifestyle, intentions, finances etc. Tends also to occur in people who have decided they are drinking too much and who try to abstain.

Bowlby, John (1907–) A leading British psychoanalyst especially famed for his report to the World Health Organisation on *Maternal Care and Mental Health*, in which the importance in the first few years of the mother and baby's **attachment** was emphasized. Subsequently, in his trilogy *Attachment and Loss*, Bowlby has reformulated psychoanalytical principles in the light of **ethology**, control theory and cognitive psychology. *See also* **hospitalism**.

brain amines With reference to biological **psychiatry** denotes **neurotransmitter** substances (noradrenaline, dopamine and serotonin). Abnormalities in the synthesis, release, re-uptake and metabolism of amines are thought to be involved in the **aetiology** of the functional **psychotic** illnesses such as **manic-depressive psychosis** and **schizophrenia**.

brain atrophy Shrinkage of brain substance due to physical processes. *See also* **dementia**.

brain damage Disease of or injury to the brain, leading to permanent anatomical and functional changes.

brain tumour An abnormal multiplication of brain cells causing a swelling that destroys or compresses healthy brain cells and increases the pressure within the skull. Benign tumours are slow-growing, while malignant tumours spread and cause progressive impairment of brain functions. Can originate in the brain (primary) or be secondary deposits from a malignant lesion elsewhere in the body.

brainwashing Techniques including indoctrination, repeated **suggestion**, mental exhaustion to produce deliberate transformation of attitudes or **personality** in pursuance of some political or other non-therapeutic aim, e.g. to extract confessions or make the prisoner adhere to the enemy's doctrines.

breath-holding attacks   Commonly occur in children between the ages of six and thirty-six months usually in response to frustration. Often initiated by persistent crying; the infant goes into a tantrum and suddenly stops breathing. Cyanosis, **unconsciousness** and more rarely an epileptiform seizure may occur. After the development of cyanosis the attack usually ends abruptly with the child taking a deep breath and, often after a further cry, returning to normal.

Brentano, Franz (1838–1917)   Viennese philosopher whose lectures **Freud** attended and who influenced **Husserl**. He emphasized that all mental acts exhibit intentionality i.e. refer to an object (e.g. a coloured surface, the concept of beauty, Aphrodite, etc.) distinct from the mental act that refers to it.

Breuer, Josef (1842–1925)   A general practitioner in Vienna who discovered the cathartic method of the treatment of hysteria, in which he interested **Freud**. Together they published *Studien über Hysterie* (1895).

Brill, Abraham A. (1874–1948)   First American psychoanalyst, early translator of Freud's works into English.

Briquet's disorder   Paul Briquet (1796–1881) was the author of a monumental treatise on hysteria (1859). In recent years his name has been attached to those who present repeatedly as patients to many clinics with numerous different bodily complaints, including pain, and in whom there is little evidence of significant physical illness and a marked tendency to chronicity.

broken home   *See* **family breakdown**

bruxism   *See* **teeth grinding**.

buggery   Usually refers to anal intercourse, either hetero- or homosexual, but in law also includes sexual contact with an animal (*see* **bestiality**).

bulimia   Gross overeating or voracious appetite. The symptoms can accompany or follow **anorexia nervosa**.

bulimia nervosa   A condition in which bouts of gross overeating (**binges**) produce feelings of bloating, nausea and malaise often followed by vomiting and purgation. It is often associated with perverse attitudes or **behaviour** related to eating and body weight, and is commonly associated with **anorexia nervosa**.

burn out   A state developing in professionals working in stressful situations, eg. **therapeutic communities** or intensive **social work** with disturbed families, in which efficiency and coping capacity deteriorate, and only improve with the move to another working environment.

burnt out   A term sometimes applied to that **residual** (or end) **state** in **schizophrenia** in which after many years of illness the patient has few florid **symptoms**, which if present are well encapsulated, and the clinical features are those of a **defect state**. These patients lack initiative, are socially withdrawn and have poor social skills. *See also* **defect state**.

Burrow, Trigant L. (1875–1951)   American psychiatrist who studied with Freud and Jung and introduced the term 'group analysis', but as group therapy developed he renamed his study of behaviour in groups as 'phylo-analysis'.

Burt, Sir Cyril (1883–1971)   Eminent British psychologist who studied educational backwardness, mental subnormality and delinquency. Posthumously discredited for misreporting his research findings.

butyrophenones   **Drugs** used as alternatives to **phenothiazines**, e.g. in the treatment of **schizophrenia**. Haloperidol is an example. Sometimes, used for the restlessness found in **organic** psychiatric illnesses such as **delirium**.

cachexia   The condition of bodily wasting caused by prolonged starvation or the ravages of chronic malignant or infective disease.

cannabis   (syn. marijuana, hashish; sl. 'hash', 'grass', 'pot', 'the weed') Parts of the hemp plant (*Cannabis sativa*), dried, containing isomers of tetrahydrocannabinol, illegally used for their psychoactive effects including an increased sense of well-being and alterations in **memory** and the sense of time. In excess, a toxic **confusional state** may occur. Contradictory data exist regarding its chromosomal damaging effects through chronic use, and its association with **psychosis** and amotivational states.

carpopedal spasm   Spasm of the hand muscles resulting in extension of the wrist with distal finger joints extended and proximal joints flexed (*main d'accoucheur*). Associated with tetany, rickets and **hysterical hyperventilation** states. The latter results in severe alkalosis which can be dramatically reversed by breathing into a paper bag.

castration anxiety

castration anxiety   Term originating in classical **psychoanalytic theory** to signify dread of loss of sexual organs especially penis in males; now elaborated to denote **fear** of deprivation or loss of potency or power in either sex, although most often referring to the consequences of humiliating domination by a more powerful person.

castration complex   Term in **psychoanalytic theory** to denote a group of interconnected **beliefs** and feelings, mostly **unconscious**, which exert recurrent effects on conscious **behaviour** and attitudes and which centre on themes concerned with **castration anxiety**.

CAT scan   *See* **computerized axial tomography**.

catalepsy   Abnormal immobility of physical posture with increased muscle tone, some **resistance** to change of posture (**negativism**), and sometimes waxy flexibility (**flexibilitas cerea**). Occurs most often, but still rarely, in **catatonic schizophrenia**, but has been found in drug-induced conditions, **encephalitis** lethargica and other brain disorders. Its cause probably includes both psychopathological and neurophysiological factors.

cataplexy   Abrupt brief loss of muscle tone, generalized or mainly in the antigravity musculature, and causing collapse to the ground without loss of **consciousness**. Attacks are usually precipitated by **emotion,** especially laughter, and they occur almost exclusively in association with **narcolepsy**.

catastrophic reaction   A sudden failure to respond in a task at a level corresponding to the performance up to then, accompanied by **anxiety**, excitement and anger that may be quite violent. A term coined by **Goldstein** based on his studies of brain-injured patients to whom this reaction is almost entirely confined.

catatonia   The rarest type of **schizophrenia** characterized by sudden unpredictable alternation from **stupor** to intense excitement, even violence. The phases usually last days and in stupor the patient may show **catalepsy**. Other signs of schizophrenia are usually present as well. Occurs seldom with improved mental hospital conditions for chronically institutionalized schizophrenic patients.

catharsis   (lit. purging) Relief from subjective psychological tension or other strong **emotion** following its release; the therapeutic benefit of **abreaction**.

cathexis   From *Besetzung* (lit. investment) which Freud used in his psychoanalytical system to refer to the endowment of objects (i.e.

persons) with an emotional charge or significance. Hence also withdrawal of cathexis, for the process of decathexis when the emotional significance of another person is reduced.

central nervous system   A general term referring to the brain and spinal cord in contrast to the peripheral nervous system which comprises the autonomic nerves and nerves in the limbs and trunk outside the cord.

cephalalgia   Headache.

cerea flexibilitas   *See* **flexibilitas cerea**.

cerebral arteriosclerosis   Atheromatous disease of brain arteries producing strokes and other physical manifestations of focal brain disease. Alternatively, or in addition, **dementia** may occur. *See also* **arteriosclerotic dementia, multi-infarct dementia**.

cerebral atrophy   *See* **brain atrophy**.

cerebral degeneration   A non-specific term encompassing loss of brain tissue, due to a wide variety of causes, such as disease or a defective blood supply.

cerebral localization   The association of specific physical or psychological functions with particular brain areas, e.g. speech with the language centre in the dominant hemisphere.

character disorder   A condition in which the fundamental abnormality is of habitual **behaviour** and attitudes; **symptoms**, if present, are of secondary importance. The problem consists of a disturbance of **personality** functioning, taking the form of an exaggeration or distortion of certain character traits. In **psychoanalysis**, character usually refers to those attributes of a person which enable him to be categorized into one of a number of character types (e.g. **oral, anal, genital**), and not to those which most categorize him as an individual person.

Charcot, Jean-Martin (1825–1893)   Great neurologist who used **hypnosis** and studied hysteria at the Saltpêtrière Hospital in Paris where he was visited by **Freud**, whom he influenced decisively. **Janet** and Binet were also his students.

Chiarugi, Vincenzo (1759–1820)   Illustrious physician to the hospital of St. Boniface in Florence. Reformer of the treatment of the insane in Italy.

child abuse   Persistent injury or damage to a child, often by a parent, close relative or guardian, most frequently of a physical nature and often motivated by conscious or **unconscious** feelings of rejection and resentment. *See also* **non-accidental injury**.

child analysis   The **psychoanalytic** treatment of children in which **play therapy** replaces **free association**. Based on **psychodynamic** principles (usually Freudian or Jungian), it differs in that parents are still actual, external figures in the patient's life, and **dependence** on them is a social and biological fact, not a neurotic symptom as in adult **analysands**.

childhood autism   *See* **early infantile autism**.

chlordiazepoxide   A **benzodiazepine drug** used in the treatment of **anxiety** states.

chromosomal sex   The sex of a fetus is determined primarily by whether the **zygote** contains two X **chromosomes** (i.e. one from each parent) which is female or an X and a Y chromosome (i.e. X from mother and Y from father) which is male. The sex chromosomes determine whether the primitive gonad develops into a female ovary or male testis. Most of sexual differentiation then stems from the hormonal consequences of this gonadal differentiation.

chromosome   The intracellular structure containing the genetic material DNA is a nucleoprotein complex, which has special staining properties, hence the term chromosome. The number in a cell is characteristic of a species. The human has 46, two of which are sex chromosomes, determining sex and other sex-linked characteristics (two X, female; X and Y, male). The other 44 are called autosomes. When a cell divides, the 46 chromosomes divide to produce two paired sets. This is called mitosis. When a gamete (ovum or spermatazoon) is formed, a special form of cell division produces a half or haploid set of 23 chromosomes. This is called meiosis.

chromosome anomalies   Two kinds of error occur during gametogenesis. Abnormalities of chromosome number result from nondisjunction, i.e. a pair of chromosomes does not separate during meiosis, leaving a gamete with one too many (trisomy) or one too few (monosomy). Such cells are called aneuploid. Abnormalities of chromosome morphology most commonly arise from translocation of one section of chromosome to another. Other abnormalities include inversion and deletion. *See also* **chromosome**; **Down's syndrome**; **sex chromosome anomalies**.

chronic Describes a state which persists over a long period of time, or permanently.

circadian rythms Biological activities following cycles that repeat at approximately 24 hour intervals.

circumstantial speech Speech not directly to the point and with ample irrelevant detail. It may be seen in **neurosis**, especially in obsessional **personality** disorder, in **schizophrenia** and **manic psychosis,** and in **confusional states** when the individual has **clouded consciousness** and impaired **orientation.**

circumstantiality A quality of speech or **behaviour** in which transient events and incidental topics carry undue influence, resulting in talk which is overdetailed, lacking in direction and marred by connected irrelevancies. Found in some healthy people and in certain immature **personalities** (e.g. **obsessionals**) and in certain illnesses (e.g. **schizophrenia**) in which the individual repeatedly strays from the point of the matter in hand.

claustrophobia Morbid **fear** of enclosed places.

climacteric The time in a woman's life when her ovarian function starts to fail, eventually leading to cessation of cyclical hormone production and menstruation (i.e. the **menopause**). A further period of adjustment occurs during which vasomotor and other symptoms are common. This whole perimenopausual period is sometimes known as the climacteric. The average age for cessation of menstruation is 50 years. The duration of the change and adjustment before and after this event varies from months to many years.

clinical psychologist *See* **psychologist**.

clouded consciousness A moderate degree of general lowering of level of **consciousness** such as is found in mild **confusional states**, and due to **organic** disturbances of brain function. For superficially similar but different disorders of consciousness *see* **dissociative state; dreamy state.**

clouding *See* **mental clouding**.

cocaine addiction Severe psychological **dependence** on the crystalline white powder derived from the leaves of *Erythroxylon coca*; often taken intranasally (snorted), it has a powerful stimulant action. Cocaine **psychosis** is characterized by **paranoid** ideas, restlessness and **hallucinations**. Resembles **amphetamine addiction**.

cognition   A general term covering all the various modes of knowing and **reasoning**, including conceiving, imagining, **remembering** and judging; the psychological processes and brain mechanisms whereby knowledge is acquired, stored and integrated. The cognitive function, one of the three aspects of mind, is contrasted with the **affect** (feeling) and with **conation** (willing).

cognitive dissonance   In information theory, the psychological discomfort arising from the contemplation of simultaneously presented and contradictory messages or **perceptions**.

cognitive therapy   This is a form of **behaviour therapy** which takes as its axiom that the patient's cognitions are material in determining his mood state (and thus reverses the conventional depressive paradigm). Beck describes the 'depressive triad' (negative thoughts about self, the world, and the future) found in depressed patients. Treatment consists of encouraging the patient to keep a diary of his depressive and anxious experiences, to relate these to the stimuli and thoughts immediately preceding the abnormal mood state, with the aim of replacing the negative constructs and interpretations with a more objective and less noxious view of self in relation to others. It can be used alone in the treatment of the milder affective disorders, and it is complementary to physical methods of treatment.

cogwheel rigidity   *See* **rigidity**.

colitis, mucous   A chronic or recurrent disorder with looseness of stool or diarrhoea, associated with colic. There is no **organic** change in the large bowel and emotional disturbance may play a part in the causation.

colitis, psychogenic ulcerative   *See* **psychogenic**.

coma   Loss of **consciousness** of considerable depth, i.e. unrousability by all stimuli, though some autonomic reflex responses to pain may be observed. The condition is nearly always **organic** in **aetiology** (**drugs**, brain disease, toxic states etc.) but the term 'hysterical coma' is sometimes used to cover profound hysterical **dissociative states** with immobility; many physical responses are then preserved.

combat fatigue   *See* **battle fatigue**.

comfort eating   (syn. compulsive eating). Eating at inappropriate times or eating unusual amounts as a consolation or for the relief of distress, depressed **mood** or **anxiety**. Often the food is of high caloric content, e.g. chocolate, loaves of bread or packets of biscuits.

community psychiatry *See* **psychiatry**.

compensation An unconscious **defence mechanism** enabling the individual to attempt to overcome or make up for real or fantasied deficiencies. The term may also be used for the conscious attempt to overcome some disability. See also **compensation neurosis**.

complex A group of related ideas and feelings, some or all of which are **unconscious**, which exerts a dynamic influence on conscious feelings, attitudes and **behaviour**, e.g. **inferiority complex, Oedipus complex**, and may result in the person thinking, feeling and acting in a **stereotyped**, repetitive way.

Electra complex A term analogous to **Oedipus complex** to denote a pathological emotional attachment, with an **unconscious** erotic attachment, of a daughter to her father or father-figure.

inferiority complex A term associated with the psychological theory of **Adler**, referring to a sense of inadequacy in relation to others and characterised by feelings of **unworthiness**, low self-esteem, abnegation, physical short-comings and social shame. The affected person by **overcompensation** may achieve high ambitions or develop special skills.

Oedipus complex **Psychoanalytic** term coined by **Freud**. It develops in both sexes between the ages of three to five years. Boys experience an intense erotic attachment to the mother and jealous resentment of the father and **siblings**. The forbidden desire for the mother generates **anxiety** and **unconscious fear** of penile castration (**castration complex**), and during the **genital stage** Oedipal **fantasies** are given up. The **Electra complex** is the female equivalent.

compulsion A recurrent action (such as repetitive washing) occurring with a subjective sense of pressing necessity to carry it out, under a feeling (such as **fear** of contamination) perceived to be part of a person's own **mind**, against which the person struggles. The acts may be carried out repeatedly in checking and rechecking. Compulsions are **obsessions** which take the form of actions.

compulsive eating A feeling of **compulsion** to eat which is unrelated to feelings of hunger or satiation. There is a subjective **resistance** to eating but experience of tension or distress if the impulse is denied.

computerized axial tomography (syn. CAT scan). A recently developed advance in X-ray diagnosis which entails readings taken through the head by means of narrow beams of X-rays through multiple projections at many different angles from a succession of transverse planes. From the data so derived, absorption values for each plane are calculated on a computer making it possible to present a picture of each anatomical transverse layer studied.

conation A term for the mental activities that lead to purposeful action (the will, **volition, motivation**, the **drives**). Separate from the other two parts of the mind, **cognition** (intellectual) and **emotion**. For abnormal aspects of conation *see* **passivity feelings; catatonia**.

concussion A transient (seconds or hours) period of unconsciousness following injury to the head. There is total **amnesia** for the accident, but following it the patient may continue quite well co-ordinated activity (e.g. playing football after being kicked). There is no recognizable structural damage to the brain, but there may be effects on a mid brain centre. On recovery there may be **personality** change if the injury was severe. *See also* **postconcussional syndrome**.

condensation Term in **psychoanalytic theory** used to denote the **unconscious** merging of two or more sets of **thoughts** or mental images to form a composite image having meanings derived from both, which then become represented in **dreams** and in **symptom** formation. Condensation is one of the characteristics of **primary process** thinking.

conditioned reflex A response acquired by learning which is dependent on related events. First described by **Pavlov** in experiments with dogs; he paired a stimulus (food causing salivation) with an accompanying stimulus (ringing of a bell), until the latter stimulus of itself evoked the response. The learned response may also result through operant **conditioning**.

conditioning Establishing new **behaviour** in ordinary experience or experimentally as a result of psychological modification of responses to stimuli. In the laboratory or clinic a stimulus not ordinarily related to the response in question is presented together with the stimulus that normally evokes the response. This is repeated until the first stimulus alone evokes the response (*see* **conditioned reflex**). *See also,* **conditioning, operant; reinforcement**.

aversive conditioning The extinction of an undesired **behaviour** by associating it with a painful stimulus. Occasionally used in the treatment of **alcoholism** (vomiting is induced by apomorphine when alcohol is given), **homosexuality, stuttering** etc.

operant conditioning A response is rewarded (or punished) each time it occurs, so that in time it comes to occur more (or less) frequently. Such positive **reinforcement** promotes the development of desired **behaviour**. e.g. a hungry animal offered a food reward for pulling a lever will in time be trained to pull the lever for food. Particularly associated with the name of **Skinner**. *See also* **behaviour therapy**.

conduct disorder A condition in which the central feature consists of **behaviour** which fails to conform to the social norms and expectations; the term is applied especially to children with anti-social **behaviour disorders**, including aggressive and destructive behaviour, and disorders involving **delinquency**.

confabulation The verbal linking of unrelated memories to produce a superficially intelligible account which has little basis in reality.

confidence trickster A swindler who habitually utilizes his facility for securing the trust of others and illegally or immorally abuses it, generally for financial gain. Sometimes a liar or an impostor; may be a feature of **personality disorder**.

conflict Clash between discordant and seemingly irreconcilable inclinations or impulses or their sources; may be conscious or **unconscious** and may lead to **anxiety**. In **psychoanalytic theory**, conflict between intrapsychic structures (e.g. **ego** or **id**) and conscious wishes is central to the development of **neurosis**.

confusion State of disorder of the **mind**, properly indicating the presence of an organic condition such as **delirium** most commonly or **dementia** occasionally.

confusional state A loose term imprecisely used for conditions of inappropriate **behaviour**, whether due to brain syndromes such as **delirium** or **dementia, intoxication, dissociation** of awareness as in hysterical **neurosis** or **epilepsy**, or excitement or **perplexity** in **psychosis**.

acute confusional state (syn. **delirium**, organic confusional state) Any disturbance of **consciousness** of sudden onset, with restlessness, **disorientation** for space, time and person, transient impairment of awareness and **illusions** or **hallucinations**, due to temporary changes in brain function, resulting from **intoxication**, infections, deficiency diseases, metabolic disorders etc.

Connolly, John (1794–1866)

Connolly, John (1794–1866) Abolished mechanical restraint of mental patients in the Middlesex Asylum at Hanwell in 1839, promoting the introduction of more humane care in mental hospitals.

conscience A person's sense of moral values, his **perception** of right or wrong, consciously experienced. Compare the **superego**, which differs from it in being partly **unconscious** and embodying imperatives to which the person does not consciously subscribe.

consciousness The state of being aware, in contrast to being asleep or in **coma**; the **perception** of what passes in a man's own **mind** (Locke); a concomitant of all **thought, feeling, volition** and sensory experience.

constitution An old medical term referring in some writings to the **genotype** only and in others to the total biological and physiological make-up of the individual. Psychiatric use mainly refers to the influence of the latter concept in relation to **personality** and illness in contrast to acquired or learned **behaviour** characteristics. *See also* **typology**.

constitutional Referring to the constitution of a person.

conversion A process by which a psychological **complex** which consists of ideas, wishes and feelings is replaced by a physical **symptom. Freud** discovered that **hysterical** physical symptoms are **psychogenic.** *See also* **ego, defence mechanism, hysterical conversion illness.**

conversion hysterical state *See* **hysterical conversion illness.**

conviction A firm and settled **belief.**

convulsions Attacks in which rhythmic uncontrollable shaking of the limbs occurs, usually associated with **coma.** Febrile convulsions are provoked by fever in children. Often part of **epilepsy,** or can occur with injury or impairment of the brain. Fits similar in appearance can be **hysterical.**

coprolagnia That sexual variation or anomaly in which sexual excitement is associated with faeces or defaecation.

coprolalia The recurrent utterance of filthy and obscene words especially those related to faeces. In association with **tics,** occurs in **Gilles de la Tourette syndrome;** also in some patients with **obsessional neurosis,** and sometimes in **schizophrenia.**

coprophagia The deliberate eating of dung or faeces. Occurs in the intellectually subnormal, in regressed **catatonia** in some **schizophrenic** patients, and in the **sexual deviation masochism**.

coprophilia An unusual interest in filth especially in faeces and in defaecation, and sometimes hoarding of faeces or dung.

Cotard's syndrome A **nihilistic delusion** which may lead the sufferer to deny his own existence and that of the outside world. Although some claim this as a distinct clinical entity it is probably best regarded as a nihilistic delusion which may occur in **depressive psychosis** or certain **organic** states.

counselling A process of consultation and discussion in the course of which one individual (counsellor) offers advice or guidance to another (client) on particular or general personal problems. One of the methods used by **psychiatric social workers**, and in other helping professions and groups such as **marriage guidance** counsellors.

pastoral counselling A form of **counselling** undertaken by ministers and priests, particularly those with special knowledge and experience of **psychotherapy**.

countertransference The **psychotherapist's** personal feelings, negative or positive, for his patient, including his **unconscious** attitudes. May adverseley affect treatment, particularly if the therapist does not become aware of his unconscious **motivations**. Can help treatment by reflecting the patient's **transference** (unconscious, irrational attitudes and **behaviour**) towards the therapist.

couvade A husband experiencing symptoms such as abdominal pain, toothache or some of the accompaniments of giving birth when his wife is pregnant. From the French for hatching.

cretinism Syndrome found following congenital or postulated early failure of thyroid function. The condition can be diagnosed by early postnatal screening. Clinically it is usually obvious by six months, the patient presenting as a placid, good-natured, mentally defective dwarf with coarse dry hair and dry skin, slow responses, hernia (especially umbilical), slow pulse and distended abdomen. The condition usually responds to thyroid therapy if initiated early enough.

Creutzfeldt disease *See* **Jakob–Creutzfeldt disease**.

crime An act, usually a grave offence, punishable by law. Criminals often have psychiatric disorders, including **mental retardation,**

criminal responsibility

> schizophrenia, depressive psychosis, epilepsy, psychopathy etc. *See also* **psychiatry, forensic; responsibility,** criminal.

criminal responsibility *See* **responsibility.**

cross dressing   Dressing in clothes designed for those of the opposite sex, generally for sexual pleasure; **transvestism.**

cross tolerance   *See* **tolerance.**

cryptomnesia   **Recall** of a forgotten experience, the subject however viewing the experience as a completely new one.

culture   The total of the shared knowledge, ideas, **beliefs** and values, transmitted to successive generations and reinforced and moulded by experience, which forms the basis of the range of activities, habits, preferences, laws and opinions characteristic of a society.

culture shock   Feelings of **isolation,** rejection and alienation experienced by an individual or social group when transplanted from a familiar to an unfamiliar **culture** e.g. from one country to another.

cunnilingus   Sexual stimulation of the female's genitalia by the partner's mouth.

cybernetics   The use of mechanical or electronic devices or concepts to provide an illuminating analogy with human brain function and the associated **behaviour.** From the Greek for governing.

dance epidemics   Epidemics of **hysterical behaviour** of a florid nature including wild contortions and bodily **convulsions.** Occurred on a grand scale in medieval times. Described by Hecker in *The Dancing Manias.*

dangerousness   A judgement which the forensic **psychiatrist** often has to make, as it materially influences courts dealing with the psychiatrically disturbed, yet is impossible to evaluate accurately, especially in a predictive sense.

Darwin, Erasmus (1731–1802)   English physician who invented a chair in which the insane could be rotated, supplementing the practice of ducking. A kind of precursor of shock therapy. Grandfather of Charles Darwin.

dasein   As used by the philosopher **Heidegger** in *Being and Time (Sein und Zeit),* refers to human presence, or being present. Openness to all things, including oneself; the essence of human being. A term used in **existentialism** to refer to the distinctive character of human existence, the capacity to become aware of one's own being at any particular time, and thereby to accept **responsibility** for what one is to become in the immediate future.

day hospital A facility offering all the psychiatric modes of treatment except overnight residence. It is satisfactory especially in urban areas where transport is simple, and when home accommodation is suitable.

death Permanent cessation of all vital functions. Stopping of the heart beat used to be the medical criterion, but now brain death is emphasized when the centres controlling breathing and other vital functions permanently cease functioning.

death instinct A concept introduced by **Freud** in 1921, but not widely accepted in **psychoanalysis**, proposing a self-destructive drive opposed by the sexual instinct which perpetually seeks a renewal of life. Still adopted by followers of **Melanie Klein** who view life as a struggle against death, with the death instinct as the most powerful human instinct. May manifest as a **repetition compulsion** with the aim to annihilate oneself.

death wishes Preoccupation or fascination with, or indulgence in, life- threatening **behaviours** with or without the conscious recognition of flirting with death. Usually understood as expressions of the **death instinct** that are displaced as **unconscious** murderous wishes directed at others.

de Clérambault's syndrome *See* **delusion, erotic; erotomania.**

defect state The chronic emotional blunting, **passivity feelings** and intellectual dullness sometimes found in the later stages of **schizophrenic** illness. Not to be confused with mental defect.

defence mechanism In **psychoanalysis**, the Freudian structural theory of **mind** postulates an **ego** or self maintaining a balance between the primitive urges of the **id**, external reality and the **superego**. When the competing demands give rise to **conflicts** which produce tension, the resulting **anxiety, guilt** or disgust may be controlled or held in check by the operation of **unconscious** mental defence mechanisms. These 'mental tricks' or 'psychological lies', according to Anna Freud (*The Ego and the Mechanisms of Defence*), include **regression, repression, reaction formation, isolation, undoing, projection, introjection**, turning against the self,

degeneration theory (obs)

> reversal, and **sublimation** or **displacement** of instinctual aims. *See also* **compensation; intellectualization; rationalization.**

degeneration theory (obs)   The view that the insane and criminals suffer from a hereditary taint, occurring in families that are degenerate morally and atavistically. *See also* **Lombroso, Moreau** and **Morel.**

déjà vu illusion   *See* **illusion.**

delinquency   Term applied to misdemeanours committed by children and young persons. In England children reach the age of **criminal responsibility** at 10 years and between 10 and 17 years are dealt with by special Juvenile Courts. In Scotland children from 8 up to 16 years (18 years if already in the system) are dealt with by a system of Children's Panels who try children's hearings. Most juvenile offences are against property (theft, breaking and entering) but some are violent; either solitary or in gangs. Often associated with parental inconsistency or rejection, or deprived neighbourhoods.

delirium   An **organic** brain syndrome resulting from direct or indirect impairment of the mental processes. It ranges from a barely perceptible fluctuation of **consciousness** with minimal **disorientation** and minor impairment of thinking through severe disruption of **thought** processes and restlessness. Although the central feature is the fluctuating level of **consciousness**, impairment or inversion of rhythms of **sleep**, and **behaviour**, emotional lability and restlessness are prominent features. There is usually a fearful **mood** with misinterpretations and **illusions**, and visual **hallucinations** are common. Coarse **tremors, myoclonus**, rapid heart beat and sweating are common accompaniments. *See also* **acute confusional state.**

> **acute delirium**   An **acute confusional state** which is short-lived, normally lasting hours or days.

> **subacute delirium**   A term used to describe a more persistent delirium. Usually less florid than acute delirium but lasting several weeks or longer. This may occur in a variety of conditions including **endocrine disorders,** chronic **intoxications** and cancer. Unlike other chronic organic syndromes the patient has fully lucid intervals and shows complete return of mental abilities on recovery.

delirium tremens (DTs)   A **psychosis**, occurring as an acute **withdrawal state** with **disorientation** in time, space or person, most frequently caused by alcoholism. *See also* **acute confusional state.**

delusion   An incorrigible false **belief**, inaccessible to reason and out of keeping with the cultural and educational background of the individual. German **psychiatrists** would stress the morbid origin of the delusion and distinguish between true delusions and delusion-like ideas. Thus a true delusion is the result of a primary delusional experience and cannot be deduced from any other experience, whereas the delusion-like idea is secondary and can be derived from some other morbid psychological experience. There is no entirely satisfactory classification of delusions according to their content.

depressive delusion A delusion which is compatible with the morbid depressed **mood**. Delusions of **guilt, unworthiness**, poverty, **nihilism, hypochondriasis** may all occur in association with depressed **affect**. *See also* **Cotard's syndrome.**

erotic delusion Delusions of love. **Erotomania** or **fantasy** love is a delusional **conviction** that a person of the opposite sex who may be virtually unknown to the subject is passionately in love with them. The 'victim' is often a person of great distinction or otherwise unattainable. In the **syndrome** of *psychose passionnelle* described by de Clérambault, the delusion comes to dominate the subject's life. Erotic delusions must be distinguished from **hallucinations** of a sexual nature.

grandiose delusion Exalted ideas of importance or power which may be associated with a **belief** that the patient is a historical character, e.g. Jesus Christ or Joan of Arc, or is of royal blood, has great inventive power or is able to control the thoughts and actions of others. Often but not invariably associated with elevated **mood**. *See also* **manic illness.**

delusion of guilt Some degree of heightened self-criticism or reproach is common in **depressive** states but may reach delusional intensity where patients become unshakably convinced of past wickedness, the commission of unpardonable sin or of having brought disgrace and ruin to their family. Such delusions may be associated with grandiose (the worst sinner in the world) or nihilistic ideas and may give rise to **delusions of persecution.**

hypochondriacal delusion Preoccupation with personal health or **symptoms** of illness may occur as a **personality** trait and is common in **depressive illness, anxiety** states and, to a lesser extent, in **schizophrenia.** Hypochondriacal delusions may develop from these anxieties or appear spontaneously. A **conviction** of incurable illness, insanity, cancer, venereal disease or other socially stigmatizing disorder may take on nihilistic qualities. 'The cancer has destroyed all my insides'; 'VD has turned my brain to water'.

litigious delusion Litigiousness is a pathological predilection for legal action, usually because of imagined slights or persecutions which may reach delusional intensity as persecutory delusions. *See*

delusional jealousy

also **paranoid illness; personality disorder, paranoid**.

nihilistic delusion A false **belief** that certain feelings, functions, organs or persons no longer exist, e.g. that the world has disappeared or a spouse is dead. Occurs in severe **agitated depressive illness** and in schizophrenic illness.

paranoid delusion The term paranoid originally meant delusional and in American usage implied the presence of **systematized delusions** with few if any other signs of disorganization. In English-speaking countries the accepted usage now is to mean persecutory, suspicious or hostile; thus a delusion of a hostile environment. *See also* **paranoid illness**.

delusion of persecution A **belief** that the patient has been singled out for special and usually hostile attention. The hostility, persecution or undue invasion of privacy may be held to come from definite people in the environment such as family, friends or neighbours or from groups such as the Freemasons, KGB or Scientologists.

delusion of reference The **conviction** that incidents and events in the outside world have a direct personal reference to the self; that people are looking at, talking about or disseminating information about oneself, or that mundane incidents have a specific and personal significance. *See also* **paranoid illness, schizophrenia**.

shared delusion A delusion which is transmitted from one person to one or more others with whom the originator is in some way intimately associated, e.g. spouse or family, in such a manner that they all come to share the same delusional **conviction**. On substantial separation of the partners the induced delusion subsides. Known as **folie à deux**, folie à trois etc. according to the size of the affected group.

systematized delusion Implies that a set of related delusions arises from one basic delusion with the remainder built up logically from this single erroneous assumption. This is in fact rare, and it is more common to find a loosely related set of delusional ideas which may have a related theme but often appear to have arisen independently.

delusion of unworthiness The individual is groundlessly convinced that he is worthless, a failure, has brought shame to his family, and so on. Similar to **delusion of guilt**.

delusional jealousy *See* **jealousy**.

delusional mood *See* **mood**.

dementia Refers to a global deterioration of **memory, intellect** and **judgement** together with blunting and impaired control of emotions and coarsening of the **personality** with decline in personal habits and standards. Intellectual impairment is normally the central feature, though not always the first to appear.

arteriosclerotic dementia Has come in recent years to be known as 'multi-infarct dementia' because the occlusion of blood vessels in the brain causing multiple infarction, rather than the atheroma of the vessels as such, is the cause of the dementing process. The clinical picture stands in some contrast to that of **senile dementia** of **Alzheimer's** disease and is characterized by the following features: onset is relatively abrupt, usually commencing soon after the last of a series of strokes; evidence of focal neurological or psychological deficits in the present or past; impairment of **memory** and intellectual functions is patchy and variable (rather than diffuse as in **senile dementia**), and long-established attitudes and talents may be preserved to an advanced stage; the course fluctuates, partly owing to episodes of **clouding** or **delirium** of variable severity and partly owing to new strokes; **personality** and **insight** may be partly preserved; there is greater lability of **mood** with tendencies to prominent depression and **anxiety** in early stages, and emotional incontinence; hypertension, **epileptic convulsions**, dizziness, headache are much more common than in **senile dementia**.

dementia in general paralysis *See* **general paresis**.

multi-infarct dementia (formerly **arteriosclerotic dementia** or cerebral arteriosclerosis). The syndrome of a progressive dementia of variable course in which a series of cerebrovascular accidents produce strokes or other evidence of focal brain disease, each associated with some degree of recovery. Depression is a common complication and even at quite an advanced stage of dementia insight is often preserved.

dementia praecox A term adapted by **Kraepelin** to describe the unitary **psychosis** in which he brought together four syndromes which previously had been regarded as distinct entities: hebephrenia, **catatonia,** dementia paranoides and the 'simple' form. The illness was named **schizophrenia** by **Bleuler** in 1911.

presenile dementia Refers to a group of primary dementias which commence before the age of 65 years. It includes **Pick's disease, Alzheimer's disease** of presenile type, **Huntington's chorea**, the **Parkinsonism**-dementia complex and the dementias associated with a substantial minority of cases of Friedreich's disease and other forms of spinocerebellar degeneration. **Jakob-Creutzfeldt disease** included until recently under this heading has now been shown to be due to a transmissible agent and is accordingly grouped with the secondary dementias. *See also* **dementia, simple presenile**.

dementia, secondary

> **senile dementia**   Dementia occurring usually after the age of 65 years due to atrophy of the brain, with loss of **memory**, gradual deterioration of **intellect** and disintegration of the **personality.** Virtually identical with **Alzheimer's disease**.

> **simple presenile dementia**   Refers to a form of progressive deterioration occurring before 65 years but without the focal neurological and psychological features of **Alzheimer's**, and **Pick's**, **disease.** Causes diagnostic bewilderment to some clinicians because of the absence of the features mentioned.

dementia, secondary   This refers to a group of dementias associated with specific causes such as vitamin B-12 deficiency, hypothyroidism, chronic hepatic disease, chronic **alcoholism, neurosyphilis, brain tumour, Jakob-Creutzfeldt disease** and punch drunk syndrome. When these causes are treatable, as in the case of hypothyroidism, the dementia may improve, although complete recovery is rare. **Multi-infarct dementia** is strictly speaking 'secondary' although it is usually classed with the primary cerebral degenerations. The 'secondary' character of the dementia can often be inferred from the clinical picture with its relatively short history, fluctuation in severity, patchiness of cognitive impairment, retention of some distinctive features of personality and the prominence of depressive symptoms. Such findings call for investigations to exclude the possibility of a primary and possibly treatable cause.

denial   In **psychoanalysis**, a **defence mechanism** by which an aspect of reality is overlooked or minimized and replaced by a wish-fulfilling self-deception, e.g. a person may deal with homosexual inclinations by a psychological posture of determined and even exaggerated masculinity (**overcompensation**).

dependence   The psychological or physical effects produced by the taking of certain **drugs**, characterized by a **compulsion** to continue taking the drug. In physical **dependence** withdrawal of the drug causes specific symptoms (**withdrawal syndrome**). *See also* **addiction**.

> **physical dependence**   A state in someone addicted to alcohol or **drugs** manifesting itself by intense physical disturbance (e.g. sweating, tremulousness) when the level of the drug in the body falls (as in 'morning shakes' with **alcoholism**). Compare psychological dependence. *See also* **withdrawal syndrome**.

> **psychological dependence**   The emotional aspect of **addiction** to a **drug**, including alcohol, when repeated usage has induced reliance on the substance for a state of well-being and psychic satisfaction. Can occur with or without physical **dependence**.

depersonalization A change in the self, consisting of an unpleasant subjective state with a pervading sense of unreality. The individual may experience observing his own body or activities in a detached fashion. There may be an accompanying sense of remoteness, artificiality and unreality of the surrounding environment (**derealization**). Depersonalization may occur in normal individuals and in a wide variety of psychiatric disorders.

depersonalization syndrome An illness, category no. 300.6 in **ICD-9,** referring to a **neurotic** disorder where **depersonalization** is the predominant feature. In **DSM-III** classified as a **dissociative** disorder because of the disturbance in the sense of one's own reality, even though **memory** is not impaired, as it generally is in other disorders in this category.

depressants Drugs which depress and decrease the activity of the **central nervous system**, resulting in lowered levels of alertness and motor response, and reduction of **mood**.

depression Sad mood, dejection, or hopelessness usually as a consequence of a disappointment in life.

depressive illness A **syndrome** of depressed **mood**, disturbed **thinking** and slowing down of mental and physical activity. The subdivision of depressive illness is commonly into neurotic or **reactive depressive illness** on the one hand and **endogenous depressive illness** on the other. **ICD-9** recognizes **manic-depressive psychosis,** corresponding to endogneous depressive illness, and neurotic depression, apparently provoked by a saddening experience. In the United States **DSM-III** includes within major **affective disorders:** bipolar disorder, depressed, when there is also a history of manic disorder, and major depression when there is not. Dysthymic disorder is the US term in **DSM-III** corresponding to neurotic depression in **ICD-9.**

agitated depressive illness A major depressive illness accompanied by severe **agitation** and restlessness. Some consider that there is no justification for regarding this as a separate diagnostic entity, for agitation may be a feature of any **affective disorder.** Seen in middle age and formerly known as involutional **melancholia** when occurring at that time.

endogenous depressive illness A depressive disorder in which constitutional factors have a major role, and biological symptoms such as early morning wakening, marked weight loss, diurnal variation of **mood** and slowing of biological functions predominate, e.g. loss of appetite, sleeplessness and absent sexual interest. **Guilt**

and self-reproach may reach delusional intensity and **hallucinations** or **delusions** in keeping with the **affective** state may develop. *See also* **reactive** (or **neurotic**) **depressive illness**.

masked depressive illness A major depressive illness in which the individual denies or conceals depression of **mood** but may present with an insistent somatic complaint, most commonly atypical **pain** in the face or head. Careful enquiry will usually elicit other depressive **symptoms**.

monopolar depressive illness A major depressive disorder corresponding to an **endogenous depressive illness** with no history of **manic illness**.

postpartum depressive illness Two or three days after childbirth many women experience a period of emotional lability in which depression and tearfulness are common, the so-called 'blues'. Neurotic depressive **symptoms** which have been present during pregnancy may be exacerbated after delivery, or depressive symptoms may arise *de novo* shortly after delivery or after a delay of some weeks. The distinction between **neurotic** or **reactive depressive illness** and **psychotic affective disorder** is of considerable significance in terms of treatment.

psychotic depressive illness A major illness in which the depressed **mood** is reflected in **delusions** or **hallucinations** which do not arise from any other pre-existing disorder.

reactive depressive illness A depression of **mood** in response to a particular event or its anticipation, which may be a loss of a loved person, or revived feelings associated with a previous loss. *See also* **neurosis, depressive**.

derealization Unpleasant subjective awareness of the environment as artificial, remote, unreal. Often occurs in association with **depersonalization** either in normal individuals or in a wide variety of psychiatric disorders.

dermatitis artefacta Injury to the skin, usually scratches, caused deliberately by the person affected, who denies that it is self-inflicted.

desensitization A type of **behaviour therapy** whereby a response is taught to the patient as a substitute for troublesome responses which the treatment seeks to reduce or remove, e.g. a person with a **phobia** for air travel can be trained in **relaxation**, or one with a dog phobia can be shown pictures of dogs, then given contact with a docile small dog, graduating to large dogs. Can be combined with **drug** treatment or **psychotherapy**.

determinism Philosophical view that free will and personal choice are illusory and that **behaviour** is the inexorable result of a chain of causes.

diathesis The tendency to develop certain disorders, e.g. tubercul(, which may run in families but are not directly inherited.

diazepam A **benzodiazepine** drug.

dietary chaos syndrome A recently introduced term intended to include patients who maintain a normal or moderately above-average weight with periods of abstinence from food alternating with periods of **bulimia.** They often employ a variety of devices such as vomiting, purgation or prolonged chewing of food without swallowing. The central preoccupation is with the notion that control of eating and weight is the key to well-being.

disorientation The state of loss of awareness of space, time or **personality.** It can result from organic brain disease in **dementia** or **delirium,** or from **drugs,** or from **anxiety.**

displacement An **unconscious** mental **defence mechanism** involving the transfer of **emotion** from the original idea or person to another which is usually less threatening, or the shifting of **id** impulses from one pathway to another. The discharge of emotion onto a less powerful object (kicking the cat instead of the boss) is of course often practised as a conscious activity.

dissociation **Defence mechanism** whereby large elements of the conscious **mind** are split off and function autonomously. There may be **repression** of one of the elements, e.g. in **fugue** states, or alternation of the elements as in multiple **personality.**

dissociative state A disturbance in the normal integration of **consciousness**, in which elements of the **mind** are split off and function autonomously (*See* **dissociation**).

distortion An absence of correspondence between **perception** of a stimulus by an individual and the way it is customarily perceived. In **psychoanalytic theory,** an ego **defence mechanism** in which perception of external reality is reshaped to suit inner preferences and requirements; it assists with **repression** and disguise of unacceptable feelings, **thoughts** and **percepts.** Occurs notably in dreaming.

parataxic distortion Illusory personification; any attitude towards any other person that is based on a distorted or imagined **perception** of that person or an **identification** of that person with e.g. parental figures. Occurs in individual **psychotherapy** when the patient projects onto the therapist an imaginary and very different person, e.g. a parent, to whom he addresses his utterances and

distractibility

  behaviour. According to **Sullivan,** this process commonly underlies misunderstandings in social relationships. Early adaptive attitudes to significant adults, developed to cope with them, persist and are inappropriately applied in personal relationships of later life.

distractibility   A rapid shifting of **attention,** making it difficult or impossible to carry on a logical conversation because of capricious changes in topic with irrelevant or minor stimuli. Frequently associated with **hypomania** or **mania.** It occurs also in **depressive** disorder and anxiety **neurosis,** and in children, rarely, in diffuse **brain damage.**

distributive analysis   *See* **psychotherapy.**

disulfiram   (Antabuse) A **drug** used in the treatment of **alcoholics** to render intake of alcohol unpleasant; given as oral or implanted deterrent.

Dix, Dorothea Lynde (1802–1887)   American crusader, internationally influential in improving the plight of the mentally ill, lobbying politicians and founding mental hospitals.

Don Juanism   (obs.) Term implying the need for a man to make numerous sexual conquests over women, and an associated difficulty in establishing or maintaining a stable sexual relationship. In psychoanalysis sometimes viewed as a defence against unconscious homosexual impulses.

dopamine *See* **brain amines**

doppelgänger   Awareness of the presence of a 'double' placed in close proximity to the subject. May include an **hallucination** of the self (**autoscopy**).

double-bind   Mutually contradictory verbal and non-verbal communication. e.g. a mother reproaching her son as timid may punish him for any show of assertiveness. Erroneously regarded by **Bateson** as a factor in the **aetiology** of **schizophrenia** when experienced repeatedly in childhood.

Down's syndrome   A congenital condition, previously called mongolism, associated with various structural abnormalities including characteristic 'mongoloid' facies and **mental retardation.** It is caused by an autosomal **chromosomal anomaly,** trisomy 21 which results either from non-disjunction (the commonest, especially in older mothers) or translocation.

dream   A series of pictures or events experienced during **sleep.** In **psychoanalytic theory**, dreams are assumed to have meaning which can be arrived at by **interpretation**: the dream as experienced is the **manifest content**; the **latent content** is discovered by the **psychotherapist's** exploration with the dreamer when awake. Dreams are more easily recovered during the five or so phases of **sleep** (REM) when rapid eye movements occur. The function of dream sleep (the **paradoxical** phase) may be to process the sensory intake of the preceding day.

dream interpretation   An ancient and almost universal practice in human societies of seeking significance in dreams. In this century dreams have been systematically studied by many **psychiatrists**, especially **Freud** and **Jung**. Patients' dreams are often routinely investigated in explorative **psychotherapy**. *See also* **latent** and **manifest content**.

dreamy state   A term first used by **Jackson** to describe a variety of **aura** experienced by some patients with temporal lobe **epilepsy.** It is sometimes wrongly used more loosely to describe any dream-like condition due to a variety of causes, e.g. **drugs, hysterical illness, psychosis**.

drive   Innate tendency in animals or humans to certain goal-directed **behaviour**, e.g. pursuit of food, sexual contact. More generally in humans, the level of psychic energy expressed as striving behaviour in many contexts. In **psychoanalysis**, two drives are distinguished, the sexual or erotic (the energy of which is the **libido**) and the destructive (the energy of which is destructiveness).

drug   Any substance that, when taken into the living organism, may modify one or more of its functions. In popular usage, **narcotic** and other addictive drugs that are used illegally.

drug abuse   Persistent or sporadic excessive drug use inconsistent with or unrelated to acceptable medical practice.

drug addiction   This term has been widely and inconsistently used to such an extent that it can no longer be used without qualification or elaboration. Some authorities advocate that it should be used to mean a pattern of compulsive drug use, characterized by overwhelming involvement with the use of the drug and the securing of its supply, with a high tendency to relapse after withdrawal. *See also* **drug dependence**.

drug dependence   A state, psychic and sometimes also physical, resulting from the interaction between a living organism and a drug, characterized by behavioural and other responses that always include a **compulsion** to take the drug on a continuous or periodic basis in order to experience its psychic effects, and sometimes to avoid the discomfort of its absence. **Tolerance** may or may not be present. A person may be dependent on more than one drug. *See also* **drug addiction**.

drug intoxication   Occurs when the influence of a drug is such that **behaviour** is influenced or **consciousness** altered or impaired, e.g. after taking excessive amounts of alcohol.

drug misuse   A term inconsistently used as a synonym for **drug abuse.** It tends to be used to include occasional pleasure-seeking drug use, persistent use of **tranquillizers** or night sedation, and if the term is to continue in use it should probably be confined to individual mild abuse independent of a group drug subculture.

drug tolerance   *See* **tolerance**.

drunkenness   *See* **alcohol intoxication**.

DSM–III   *Diagnostic and Statistical Manual of Mental Disorders,* Third Edition, prepared by the Task Force on Nomenclature and Statistics of the American Psychiatric Association, 1980.

Durkheim, Emil (1858–1917)   French sociologist who was a founder of modern sociological method. He wrote *Le Suicide* (1897), identifying one contributing factor as **anomie**, the weakening of shared social values and **beliefs** in a **culture**. Such loss of the cohesive forces in society favours an increase in the **suicide** rate.

dwarfism   Pathologically small stature, either **genetic** in origin, or due to secondary deformity of limbs or spine, or of **endocrine** nature, or due to malabsorption of food or other metabolic disorders; frequently associated with infantilism.

pituitary dwarfism   Small stature with absence of sexual hair and underdeveloped sex glands and adrenal glands, due to deficiency of pituitary gland function. No known cause in the majority of cases, but a **genetic** defect may be responsible for some. Acquired forms follow damage to the pituitary gland by tumours, **meningitis** or injury.

psychosocial dwarfism   Growth retardation (height and weight) in infants and children exposed to persistent neglect or hostility by their caretakers where no other organic cause for the retardation can be found. Often accompanied by failure of emotional and social development. Both psychological responsiveness and physical growth improve when the children are placed in a nurturing environment.

dyadic   Relating to a pair; concerned with the interactions between the two individuals comprising a couple. *See also* **psychotherapy**.

dying   The process leading to death during which the individual is anticipating his impending demise. Emphasized in **existential psychiatry,** where a person's existence is a being-toward-death. Awareness of dying is a distinctively human characteristic. In inauthentic living the person defends himself from awareness of the inevitability of dying by diversion, **denial** and other self-deceiving devices. *See also* **thanatology**.

dynamics   The forces or variables that produce movement or change in a field or system. In **psychology** and **psychiatry**, concerned with environmental and intrapersonal influences which determine the course of psychological development, and with the study of emotional processes and **motivation.** e.g. **Psychoanalysis** is a dynamic psychology, in that its concepts of process and development imply movement; the contrast is with the static psychologies which define attributes of the **mind.** *See also* **psychodynamic**.

dynamism   Term used by **Sullivan** to denote habitual patterns of **behaviour** and of relating to others. A persisting pattern of interpersonal behaviour. Conjunctive dynamisms bring people together and disjunctive dynamisms drive them apart.

dysarthria   Disordered articulation of speech, due to drugs or to lesions or damage to the musculature, its nerve supply, or centres of the brain which modulate and integrate the muscles connected with speech.

dyscalculia   A specific relative inability to deal with numerical problems at the level compatible with the person's mental age and level of performance of other cognitive functions such as reading or writing. It has been ascribed to a focal lesion in the parieto-temporal area of the dominant side of the brain.

dysgenesis   Abnormal development usually applied to embryological failure (*See* **dysgenesis, gonadal**).

gonadal dysgenesis   Abnormal development of the testes or ovaries resulting in deficient or absent gonadal tissue. In both **genetic** males and females the physical development is along female lines until past the age when **puberty** normally occurs. In the case of the genetic male, female development occurs because of lack of Mullerian inhibiting factor and testosterone. **Turner's syndrome** is a special form of gonadal dysgenesis due to a missing **X chromosome**, *see* **XO syndrome**.

dyskinesis Abnormal movements usually applied only to activity of limb and face but can be more generally applied to all movements (e.g. from lesions of the basal ganglia in the brain). Includes chorea, dystonia and the involuntary movements occurring as side effects with **phenothiazine drugs**.

dyslalia A defect of articulation of speech in which consonants are omitted or substituted for each other, in the absence of abnormalities of the musculature or of its range of possible movements. It is commonly associated with **mental retardation** but also occurs in the psychologically disturbed child as a symptom of **regression**.

dyslexia Difficulty in recognition of the written word, often caused by neurological dysfunction, occurring in the school child; merges with more common reading difficulties based on faulty **learning**.

dysmnesia Any disturbance of **memory**, usually involving defects of retention or **recall**. Various forms occur depending mainly on the cause which may be **psychogenic** (i.e. posthypnotic) or more commonly **organic** as in **Korsakoff psychosis**.

dyspareunia Pain or discomfort experienced by the woman during actual or attempted sexual intercourse. Psychological or physical causes may be responsible. *See also* **vaginismus**.

dysphagia Difficulty in swallowing.

dysphagia globosus or dysphagia hysterica Synonyms for **globus hystericus**.

dysphasia *See* **aphasia**.

dysphonia A disorder of speech due to dysfunction of the vocal chords producing hoarseness or other impairment of voice production.

dyspraxia A high level disturbance of voluntary motor activity in which complex purposeful movements or groups of movements (e.g. gesturing, opening a matchbox) are impaired. The disorders are related to lesions of the cerebral cortex of the brain, and lower level disorders (muscular weakness or inco-ordination or sensory changes) if present are minor and insufficient to account for the patient's inability to organize the movements.

dysthymic disorder   *See* **depressive illness**.

early infantile autism   A childhood **psychosis** consisting of **autistic withdrawal** (characterized by gaze-avoidance), absent or abnormal language development (characterized by **echolalia** or parroting), and **obsessional** repetitive behaviours, all beginning under the age of 30 months. *See also* **autism**.

eating disorders   A group of disorders in which there is an abnormal attitude to or preoccupation with eating and or body weight. These include **anorexia nervosa, bulimia nervosa, compulsive eating, dietary chaos syndrome, pica, psychogenic vomiting** and overeating.

echo reactions   Repetitive imitation by the patient of speech or movements of another person.

manneristic echo reactions   Echo reactions stamped with an idiosyncratic quality.

echolalia   Continual repeating of that which is being said to one by another instead of replying. It is a **mannerism** associated with **anxiety** but in the most striking forms is a feature of **schizophrenia** or **brain damage**.

echopraxia   Morbid imitation of the actions of others. *See also* **latah**.

ecology   Study of the mutual relationship between individuals and their environment. In **psychiatry** it concerns the distribution of mental disorders in defined populations in relation to social and other factors. *See also* **psychiatry, social**.

ECT   *See* **electroconvulsive therapy**.

ectomorph   A body type characterized by Sheldon, consisting of a long thin physique, associated by him with solitariness and social withdrawal. *See* **endomorph, mesomorph, typology**.

EEG   *See* **electroencephalogram**

effeminacy   **Behaviour** in males reminiscent of female styles. Conspicuous in some male homosexuals.

ego   In **psychoanalysis** the part of the **mind** which is in relation to the external world, governed by the **reality principle** and **secondary processes**, and hence realistic, adaptive, ensuring self-preservation, and aware of and responsive to the demands of the environment. The task of the ego is to mediate between the forces of these unconscious psychological structures and reality. The **defence mechanisms** are psychological processes such as **denial** by which the ego protects against unacceptable or socially damaging impulses from the **id**.

weak ego   An ego structure lacking the capacity to integrate **id**, **superego** and reality forces, and hence unable to mediate requirements for adaptive responses to inner and outer pressures on the individual.

ego-alien   In classical **psychoanalytic theory** the **id**, which serves as the locus of instinctual **drives** governed by the **primary process**, is developmentally prior to the **ego** and therefore ego-alien. The concept of **dissociation** postulates that aspects of the self which are in **conflict** with the ego are repressed and continue to operate outside awareness; such self-components are then ego-alien, e.g. homosexual inclinations in an overassertively heterosexual person.

eidetic image   A vivid image, visual or auditory, experienced not as in the **mind** but projected into the environment, with the clarity of real **perception.** After examining a picture for a few seconds some normal children on looking at a grey screen report that they can see it again, and are able to describe it in minute detail. The basis of capacity for such eidetic imagery is unknown; it diminishes in adulthood and has no known psychological significance.

elective mutism   *See* **mutism**.

Electra complex   *See* **complex**.

electroconvulsive therapy (ECT)   A form of treatment used mainly for highly selected cases of severe **depressive illness**, in which the patient is caused to experience a series of electrically induced **convulsions.** A course of treatment generally consists of five to eight applications, over a 3 or 4-week period. Newer ECT machines deliver high voltage in very brief DC pulses with less electrical energy being passed across the brain than with older apparatus. Unilateral electrode placement is now regarded as preferable to bilateral placement, causing less memory disturbance. The effects of the shock are modified by the previous administration of intravenous anaesthetic and muscle relaxant. Scrupulous attention is required to technical details and to assessment and supervision of the patient.

electroencephalogram (EEG) The tracing obtained on moving paper by recording the electrical potential difference between selected points on the surface of the skull or between any of these points and a neutral reference electrode. Although it is a relatively crude summation of the more complex potentials on the surface and within the brain, it has the advantage over other forms of investigation in that it entails neither risk nor discomfort for the patient. The normal EEG is dominated by an alpha rhythm of eight to thirteen cycles per second (mainly in the occipital and parietal regions) which decreases in amplitude on opening of the eyes and is seen at maximal amplitude when the eyes are closed under resting conditions. The other rhythms are delta at less than 4 c/s, theta at 4–7 c/s, and beta at a frequency greater than 13 c/s. Localized brain lesions including epileptic foci are associated with focal discharges or asymmetrical records. Generalized impairments of **consciousness** (including those associated with **epilepsy**) arising from disturbed functioning of the diffuse **reticular formation** give rise to bilaterally synchronous symmetrical discharges.

Ellis, Havelock (1859–1939) A pioneer of sex research whose books were banned in the United Kingdom through most of his lifetime. A medical graduate, he never practised but became a major literary figure and an authority on psychological problems involving sexual behaviour. **Freud** acknowledged his debt to Ellis.

EMI scan *See* **computerized axial tomography**.

emotion Current usage equates emotion with **affect** or consciously perceived feelings together with the accompanying physical changes. Emotions are usually described in literary terms, and may be classified by their strength and breadth. The borderline between normal and pathological emotion is arbitrary.

emotional bonding The formation of lasting affectional attachments to specific figures (usually parents) during the course of development, particularly in infancy. *See also* **bonding**.

empathy The ability to recognise and identify with the subjective experience of another person; to grasp accurately and with sensitivity another person's **thoughts**, feelings and **behaviour.** In a **psychotherapist**, a necessary attribute for the treatment to succeed.

encephalitis Inflammation of the brain substance, caused by a virus or bacterium or as an allergic response. Postencephalitic **Parkinsonism** can be a complication.

encephalopathy A non-specific term meaning diffuse disease or damage of the brain affecting its function, e.g. a complication of liver disease, alcoholism etc.

encopresis The involuntary passing of faeces in inappropriate situations, starting in childhood usually after a period of normal bowel control. It may be related to constipation and 'overflow incontinence'. It is not uncommon in **mental retardation**, though in these persons control has sometimes never been obtained. Most commonly it is unassociated with any physical disorder and appears to be purely psychological in origin.

encounter therapy A form of lay group **psychotherapy** claimed to be effective treatment for personal feelings of **isolation** and alienation, in which groups of 8–18 people seek close emotional and intellectual contact by direct confrontation and frank and spontaneous expression of **thoughts** and feelings, sometimes involving bodily touch and movement.

endocrine disorders **Syndromes** of illness caused by increased or decreased activity of the ductless glands (pituitary, thyroid, parathyroid, pancreas, adrenals, gonads, thymus, pineal).

endogenous Applied to **functional** psychoses with a strong constitutional basis where external factors are absent or merely precipitating, e.g. **manic-depressive illness** and **schizophrenia**.

endomorph Body type described by Sheldon, with round physique, held by him to be associated with a relaxed outlook and sociability. *See* **ectomorph, mesomorph, typology**

engram A **memory** trace theoretically viewed as physically stored in the brain, by an alteration of the tissues.

entropy In Freudian **psychology** a loss of plasticity in redistribution of **cathexes.** This is associated with advancing years.

enuresis Involuntary passage of urine continuing after the age of normal bladder control or starting afresh after control has been established. Bed-wetting is commoner in boys than in girls and is rarely associated with any **organic** lesion of the urinary tract or **central nervous system.** Can be treated by **psychotherapy, behaviour therapy** (pad and buzzer) or **tricyclic antidepressant drugs**.

epidemiology The scientific study of the frequency and distribution of morbid states in defined populations and of the factors relating thereto.

epigenesis From embryology, where at each stage the fetus has a crucial time of development or danger of distortion. In **psychiatry** 'anything that grows has a *ground plan*, and ... out of this ground plan the *parts* arise, each part having its *time* of special ascendancy, until all parts have arisen to form a *functioning* whole' (E.H. Erikson).

epilepsy A chronic condition due to episodic disturbance of brain function, characterized by recurrent attacks, **fits** or **convulsions;** often with sudden loss of **consciousness**, with or without stiffening (tonic) and then twitching (clonic) contraction of the muscles. *See also* **epilepsy, grand mal** and **petit mal**.

absence epilepsy Very brief (2–15 seconds) impairment of **consciousness** due to generalized epileptic discharges. *See also* **epilepsy, petit mal**.

dementia epilepsy (obs.) **Dementia** formerly regarded as due to repeated **epileptic seizures.** The mental deterioration found in a few persons with epilepsy has a variety of causes and symptomatic appearances.

focal epilepsy (syn. Jacksonian epilepsy) A variant of **grand mal epilepsy** described by **Jackson**. When commencing in the motor cortex which there is a **convulsion** beginning with contraction of muscles in one area of the body, increasing in severity and spreading to involve other muscle groups, first on the same and then on the other side of the body as the attack progresses. Due to disease process in the brain cortex. In addition to such muscular forms, the 'march' can be spreading of changes in sensation (cutaneous form).

grand mal epilepsy (syn. major epilepsy, epileptic convulsion) A tonic-clonic **epileptic seizure.** The patient loses **consciousness** and falls to the ground with his muscles first in a state of spasm, and subsequently convulsive movements when the tongue may be bitten; urinary incontinence is common. Often the attack is preceded by a warning or **aura;** it can be followed by post-epileptic phenomena such as **sleep** or **confusion**.

idiopathic epilepsy Epilepsy of unknown origin, not associated with structural damage to the brain. Attacks can be of **grand mal** or **petit mal** type, and can be controlled by various **anticonvulsant drugs**.

Jacksonian epilepsy *See* **epilepsy, focal**.

petit mal epilepsy Brief spells of unconsciousness ('absences') in which posture is maintained, the eyes staring. There may be sudden spasms of the limbs, such as lifting and bending of the arms (**myoclonus**). The **electroencephalogram** shows a spike-and-wave pattern.

psychomotor epilepsy (**temporal lobe epilepsy**) A partial **epileptic seizure** usually of origin in the temporal lobe of the brain, characterized by involuntary, more or less co-ordinated motor activity with **confusion** and **amnesia.** Can be associated with **déjà vu, automatisms, hallucinations** and **illusions.** *See also* **temporal lobe epilepsy.**

status epilepsy (syn. status epilepticus) Repeated **epileptic seizures** (usually of **grand mal** type) without an intervening recovery of full **consciousness. Petit mal** can also occur producing a fluctuating **confusional state.**

temporal lobe epilepsy Strictly, epileptic attacks beginning from lesions in the temporal lobe of the brain. They are usually of **psychomotor** type but may also become generalized (**grand mal**).

epileptic aura *See* **aura.**

epileptic convulsion *See* **epilepsy, grand mal.**

epileptic fit *See* **fit.**

epileptic fugue *See* **fugue.**

epileptic furor (obs.) Rage or violence related to an epileptic attack, nearly always in a **confusional state** following a **fit.**

epileptic major fit *See* **epilepsy, grand mal.**

epileptic minor fit Any non-convulsive non-generalized epileptic attack. *See also* **epilepsy, petit mal.**

epileptic personality *See* **personality.**

epileptic prodrome *See* **prodrome.**

epileptic psychosis *See* **psychosis.**

epileptic seizure Usually a generalized **grand mal** attack but may be loosely used to refer to any epileptic attack. Seizures may also be of non-epileptic origin (e.g. hypoxia) consisting of sudden transitory abnormal phenomena such as impaired **consciousness** and other brain disburbances.

epileptic twilight state   *See* **twilight state**.

epiloia   (syn. Tuberose sclerosis) An inherited condition in which the brain, body organs and skin of the child have multiple small tumour nodules, often resulting in severe **mental retardation, epilepsy** and a 'butterfly rash' on either side of the nose.

Erikson, Erik H. (1902–)   Trained in **psychoanalysis** in Vienna, emigrated to the United States in 1933. Proposed an influential theory of the life cycle, based on an interplay between biological **epigenesis** and social challenges at different ages, with progressive unfolding of polarities (eg. basic trust vs, mistrust; industry vs inferiority) through eight epochs in succession from birth to old age. Has influenced historical research, through works such as his books on Luther and on Gandhi.

erogenous zone   (syn. erotogenic zone) A part of the body which is particularly responsive to touch during sexual stimulation. Typically, the sexual organs and the mucous membrane around body openings.

erotomania   (syn. de Clérambault's syndrome) Obsolete term for a **psychotic** state, mainly affecting women, characterized by a **delusion** that a man (often socially prominent and older) is enamoured of the patient. When shaken in their belief, some patients become amorously deluded about another man.

ESP   *See* **extrasensory perception**.

Esquirol, Jean-Etienne-Dominique (1722–1840)   French psychiatrist. Worked with **Pinel** at the Salpêtrière Hospital in Paris, giving the first series of lectures in psychiatry in 1817. He accepted the theory of cerebral localization of **Gall**, was concerned with reform of the asylums of France, and grasped the relation of social disruption and isolation to mental illness.

ethology   The observation, description and **interpretation** of the **behaviour** of animals and humans in their natural habitats.

euphoria   A transient subjectively pleasant **affective** state that seems incongruous with the patient's real life situation. Often used to indicate the effect of mild **drug intoxication** with, for example, alcohol or **amphetamine**.

excessive drinking   Misuse of alcohol, short of alcohol **addiction,** leading to harm to the person or to others. Many excessive drinkers proceed to develop alcoholism.

exhibitionism   The tendency to display one's body to others, usually display of the erect penis to a passing female. As indecent exposure, it is a common form of sexual offence, more or less confined to males; sexual excitement often occurs, but no closer physical contact is sought. Offenders brought to court show a high rate of **recidivism.** The determinants of this **behaviour** are not fully understood.

existential psychiatry   *See* **psychiatry**.

existentialism   A philosophical movement, originating with **Kierkegaard** and **Nietzsche** and then developed by **Husserl, Heidegger** and **Sartre**. Particularly influential in the years following World War II. Developed in **psychiatry** and **psychology** by **Merleau-Ponty, Jaspers, Binswanger** etc. The essential ideas point to the solitude of the individual and the ultimately subjective nature of experience and **judgement.** Since there are no objective standards and guides to ethical or other personal **behaviour**, the individual may, and must, actively choose his own path. He is responsible for the consequences of his actions. This 'doing' in the daily world determines what he 'is', as opposed to more traditional philosophical notions that 'essence' (what one is) determines 'becoming' or 'existence' (what one does). Furthermore, the constant difficult choices of existence are made against the background of the awareness of the inevitability of death. The **anxiety** of making choices is rendered the more absurd by the ultimate 'nothingness' beyond life and subjective experience. The repertoire of a person's choices is restricted by where and when one is born or unavoidably finds oneself ('Geworfenheit' or 'thrownness'). Subjectivity is free-ranging and escapes the boundaries of objective fact or judgement. The existence in the world ('Dasein') one makes for oneself should reflect the individual's subjectivity and be 'authentic', and should not be a response to what 'they', the others, either individual or institutional, expect. An existence shaped to external demand is 'inauthentic' or 'in bad faith'.

extrapunitive   Denotes a style of psychological defensive attitude whereby subjective tension and **anxiety** are held to be caused by others, or forbidden **unconscious** impulses are attributed to others against whom action can be taken to relieve personal tension.

extrapyramidal reaction   *See* **Parkinsonism**.

extrapyramidal syndrome   Disorder of that part of the brain concerned with posture, tone and the fine control of movement.

extrasensory perception (esp) As the name implies, ESP refers to unproven abilities of some persons to be aware of information (in the broadest sense) by means other than through the usual senses.

extraversion **Behaviour** which is outward-looking, sociable, gregarious. May be the habitual style in the extravert **personality**.

Eysenck, Hans Jurgen (1916–) Professor of Psychology, University of London and founding Editor of *Behaviour Research and Therapy*. A prolific researcher whose studies and writings have influenced theories of **personality disorder**, politics, **genetics** and **behaviour therapy**. He investigated the **extraversion-introversion** and the neuroticism-stability dimensions in **personality**.

factitious disorder Physical or psychological symptoms that are produced by the individual and are under voluntary control. Occurs in severe **personality disorder**. Drugs may be taken or wounds inflicted to simulate illness, e.g. causing abscesses by injecting dirt under the skin. To be differentiated from **malingering** which is undertaken with a goal in view, e.g. to evade military duty. *See also* **Munchausen syndrome**.

factitious lesions Self-inflicted damage to organs, usually cuts and scratches of the skin (*see* **dermatitis artefacta**), which the person characteristically denies having inflicted voluntarily.

factor analysis A statistical technique which extracts any tendency for variables derived from populations to cluster, thus suggesting patterns of commonality in the population.

faint A less technical term for an attack of transient loss of **consciousness** (syncope) and some other states of unsteadiness or light-headedness, often due to reduced cerebral circulation. Also occurs as a symptom of hysterical **neurosis**.

family breakdown Parent loss through death, separation, divorce or illegitimacy. The most serious and common source of privation and anxiety for young children.

family studies Investigation of psychological disorder in the family context from the viewpoint of **genetic** influences or those of the familial environment.

family therapy Psychotherapeutic process in which the therapist treats several members of the family simultaneously. 'Illness' of the individual is conceptualized as an expression of an interpersonal disorder within the family.

fantasy (phantasy) An imagined sequence of events or mental images, e.g. daydream, **masturbation** fantasy. The imaginative activity that underlies **thought**, feeling and action. In **psychoanalysis, unconscious** fantasies are held to underlie overt **behaviour**; **symptoms** of **neurosis** can be the distorted symbolic expression given to such fantasies; in **dreams**, latent dream fantasies are converted into the manifest dream scenario.

fear A feeling of apprehension associated with a real cause, or threatening person or dangerous object. The term is generally used when the emotional state is appropriate to external circumstances. Accompanying physical changes include faster heart rate, sweating, increased blood pressure etc. The accompanying **behaviour** usually is flight, submission or concealment.

feeble-mindedness In the UK, equivalent to mild **mental retardation** but in the US (and often colloquially) refers to all persons with mental handicap.

feeling *See* **affect; emotion**.

fellatio Sexual stimulation of the penis by the partner's mouth.

feral child A child found apparently having been brought up in 'the wild', following separation from human parents, thus lacking language and other human capacities, e.g. the Wild Boy of Aveyron.

festination A particular gait, seen in **Parkinsonism**, where the trunk is inclined forwards and small rapid steps are taken.

fetal alcohol syndrome. Mental and physical abnormalities due to maternal alcohol intake during pregnancy. Expectant mothers are strongly advised not to drink.

fetish An object endowed with a special sexual significance which acts as a sexual stimulus for certain people. Most commonly an article of clothing (*see* **transvestism**) or a specific texture (e.g. latex rubber) if inanimate; if animate, the preferred non-sexual parts are typically feet or hair.

fetishism The reliance on the use of a fetish object as an important or principal source of sexual stimulation.

fit   A sudden attack, as in **epilepsy**, but also colloquially of ordinary activity or **behaviour**, e.g. laughter.

epileptic fit   (syn. ictus) A loose term usually meaning generalized **convulsions** but sometimes used to refer to all epileptic attacks.

rum fit   **Epileptic seizure** due to **withdrawal** of alcohol.

uncinate fit   Strictly, an **epileptic** attack originating in the uncus of the brain, but loosely and incorrectly applied also to epileptic **dreamy states**.

fixation   A concept arising from **psychoanalysis**, which postulates that **personality development** involves specific steps to ultimate mature human heterosexuality. Various emotional and interpersonal circumstances can make progress through the necessary steps difficult, and arrested sexual and aggresive impulses are then at less mature stages.

flagellation   The use of beating, with an object such as a whip, or the hand, as a form of sexual stimulation. An aspect of **sadomasochism**.

flexibilitas cerea   (lit. waxy flexibility) Refers to the passive acceptance by a **psychotic** patient of positions imposed on his limbs, and the maintenance of these positions for periods beyond the normal limits of tolerance.

flight of ideas   The rapid movement of ideas and speech from one fragmentary topic to another that occurs characteristically in **manic** patients, the links between topics being determined by chance associations, and usually just comprehensible while far-fetched, and at times amusing.

flooding   A term used to describe the treatment approach to **phobias** in which the patient is directly presented with the feared stimulus as vividly and powerfully as possible; contra-desensitization. e.g. a patient with a morbid fear of snakes (ophidiophobia) may be taken to the large reptile house at a zoo.

folie à deux   A shared **delusion** common to two closely associated people. Characteristically the first affected is the dominant partner, the pair are comparatively isolated and the induced delusion disappears when the pair are separated.

follow-up examination   Repeated clinical assessment following discharge from hospital, or from a period of initial treatment in out-patient setting.

forensic psychiatry

forensic psychiatry *See* **psychiatry**.

foreplay The touching or caressing by sexual partners that precedes vaginal intercourse.

forgetting The normal processes of loss of memories of most of past experiences. Many factors cause forgetting, of which simple decay is probably the least important. Some apparently forgotten memories can be revived by psychological intervention, e.g. **hypnosis, free association**, drug-assisted **abreaction** ('truth drug'), **dream interpretation** etc.

formication An abnormal sensation as of insects (Latin: *formicae,* ants) crawling in or under the skin; a form of **paraesthesia.** Occurs in **functional mental illness** but is also caused by **narcotic** and other **drugs**, e.g. **cocaine** (hence 'cocaine bug'), morphine, alcohol.

fortification spectra Visual disturbances occurring in the early phase of a **migraine** attack. Commonly an expanding scintillating figure, which is coloured and angular, in the same half of the field of vision of both eyes.

free association An essential technique of **psychoanalytic psychotherapy.** The patient (**analysand**) speaks aloud his flow of ideas with as little voluntary control of the material as possible. The content, quality, errors, and patterns of this uncensored communication are thought to express **unconscious** needs, defences and **conflicts**, and are the raw material on which the analyst bases **interpretations.** The basic rule of such psychotherapy is that the patient should report his **thoughts** without reservation and make no attempt to concentrate while doing so.

Freud, Anna (1895–1982) Born in Vienna, the daughter of **Sigmund Freud**. A teacher and exceptionally gifted lay analyst. Author of *The Ego and the Mechanisms of Defence.* Developed play therapy and the **psychoanalysis** of children and adolescents.

Freud, Sigmund (1856–1939) The great Austrian neurologist and psychiatrist who founded **psychoanalysis**. He developed the concept of the dynamic structure of **mind** with **id, ego** and **superego. Libido, regression, repression, sublimation, transference**, the **Oedipus complex**, the **psychopathology** of **dreams** and everyday life, and the significance of infantile experience are all derived from his work. His influence has been great on literature, the arts and world culture, over and above his vast and revolutionary effect on **psychiatry** and **psychology**. He wrote extensively and vividly, his books widely read by the general public as well as by scholars in many intellectual disciplines.

frigidity   (obs.) Term for sexual unresponsiveness of women, and sometimes sexual revulsion.

hysterical frigidity (obs.)   Sexual unresponsiveness due to psychological impairment of **hysterical** type.

frontal lobe syndrome   A state of psychological disinhibition often with **euphoria** or grandiose **mood**, following damage to or disease of the frontal lobes of the brain.

fugue   An hysterical **dissociative state** in which the individual abruptly leaves his normal place and activity and wanders or engages in uncharacteristic **behaviour** for which he subsequently has a total **memory** loss. Often precipitated by an acute emotional setback.

epileptic fugue   An **automatism**, usually long-lasting (hours or days) in a post-ictal state (following generalized or psychomotor seizures) or, rarely, accompanying non-convulsive status epilepticus.

functional   Of a disorder which has no known physical basis. An outmoded term as applied to e.g. **schizophrenia** and **affective psychosis** which have an organic aspect although no change in structure can be demonstrated. cf **organic**.

Galen, Claudius Galerius (129–199).   Greek physician whose works marked the end of the classic Greco-Roman period of medicine and were characterized by scientific eclecticism. His medical system under the name Galenism dominated the world of medicine until the mid-eighteenth century. It was he who rejected the idea of the wandering uterus as a cause of **hysterical** illness.

Gall, Franz Joseph (1758–1828)   The founder of phrenology. Early career as anatomist whose special interest in the nervous system led him to attempt to correlate traits of **personality** with the shape of the skull in the belief that it reflected the anatomy of the underlying brain. Increasingly extravagant claims discredited what was originally a serious study but became a pseudoscience.

Gamblers Anonymous   An organization to assist compulsive gamblers, set up in 1957 in the US and in 1964 in the UK, offering group association akin to **Alcoholics Anonymous.** Members are helped with advice about settling with creditors and devising repayment arrangements. Gam-Anon is the associated body for spouses.

gambling

gambling   May be any course of risk or uncertainty but usually describes the staking of money on a chance event. Reckless gambling may occur symptomatically in a number of mental disorders, such as **hypomania.** The term **compulsive** gambling has been applied to those individuals who are unable to control their impulsive gambling **behaviour** and dissipate funds far beyond their own resources. There is no evidence of overt psychiatric illness in most such individuals. **Behaviour therapy** has been used as treatment. **Suicide** is a complication.

gamma amino butyric acid (GABA)   **Neurotransmitter** concerned in maintenance of posture, tone, and in the experience of anxiety. A degeneration of neurones which synthesize GABA occurs in **Huntington's chorea.**

Ganser, Sigbert J.M. (1853–1931)   German psychiatrist who in 1898 described a **syndrome**, frequently seen in individuals accused of crimes and awaiting trial. *See also* **Ganser state**.

Ganser state   The central feature is approximate, absurdly wrong answers to questions, together with other features such as altered **consciousness,** impaired grasp, defective **attention** and concentration, a **memory** defect, **anxiety, perplexity, hallucinations** and manifestly **hysterical** motor and sensory symptoms. Originally described in prisoners and **hysterical** in origin, it may also be found in association with organic brain impairment or serious psychiatric illness **(psychosis).** *See also* **pseudodementia, hysterical**.

gargoylism   A somewhat outmoded term for a typical coarsening and thickening of the face, associated with an inborn defect of metabolism leading to deformity of the bones, congenital corneal opacities, enlargement of the liver, and **mental retardation** (Hurler's syndrome).

geloplegia   *See* **narcolepsy**.

gender identity   Sense of maleness or sense of femaleness; a psychological state, consisting of the **conviction** usually established as early as the first three years of life that one belongs to the male or the female sex.

gender role   **Behaviour** which is a manifestation of an individual's **gender identity**, i.e. expressing masculine or feminine characteristics.

gender role disorder   Problem associated with an individual's sense of masculinity or femininity. Most commonly manifested as **behaviour** and manner which for a male is regarded as effeminate, or for a female as masculine; more rarely as **trans-sexualism.** Gender role is established largely in accordance with the sex to which an infant is assigned and reared. Separate from **sexual identity,** which is biologically determined.

gene   The functional unit of heredity. Genes are found in pairs in a constant position on a **chromosome**, and exert their effect through coding for particular protein synthesis in the cell.

   autosomal genes   The **genes** carried on non-sex **chromosomes.**

   dominant gene   A gene requiring to be present only singly (and not paired) for expression of the characteristic which it controls.

   recessive gene   A gene which only manifests its effect when both of the chromosomal pair are similar. A recessive gene does not find expression if paired with a **dominant gene.**

   sex-linked gene   A gene on the **X** chromosome which determines recessive traits, e.g. red-green colour blindness.

general paresis   Brain disorder which commences insidiously and late as a manifestation in **neurosyphilis**, with emotional lability, physical malaise, headache, disinhibition and coarsening of the **personality**, together with other features of a **frontal lobe syndrome** that may find expression in some conspicuous form of grandiose or **antisocial behaviour.** Progressive impairment of **memory** and slowing of mental activity may be punctuated by episodes of **delirium, epileptic fits** or attempted **suicide.** The condition is now very rare, and depressive paranoid forms have largely replaced the grandiose **syndromes** so prominent in the old descriptions. Gradually gives way to **apathy**, inertia and emotional emptiness in a setting of progressive physical enfeeblement, often accelerated by attacks of unconsciousness. Distinctive physical signs are present in over 90% of cases. They comprise unequal, irregular pupils sluggish in reaction or unresponsive to light, dysarthria with tremour of lips, tongue and limbs and in advanced cases, spastic paraplegia. Serological tests for syphilis are positive in blood and CSF in a great majority of untreated cases.

genetic   1. Pertaining to **genes.** 2. Produced or determined by a gene or combination of genes. 3. Pertaining to origins, history or development. 4. When combined with a noun, denotes 'pertaining to origin' or 'genesis', as in **psychogenic.**

genetic counselling

genetic counselling The process of support of and giving advice to persons for whom there is a risk that any children born to them will suffer from a genetically transmitted disorder. Sometimes adoption may be preferable (*see* **Huntington's chorea**), or antenatal diagnosis by amniocentesis may be offered. Counselling depends upon knowledge of probability of transmission found empirically and derived from information about genetic mechanisms.

genetics The science that deals with heredity.

genital stage Stage of **psychosexual** development in **psychoanalytic theory,** characterized by the organization of the instincts under the primacy of the genital zones. This organization is dominant twice: first during the **phallic stage** (infantile genital organization, ages four to six years, when the **Oedipus complex** occurs), and again at **puberty** (when the genital organization proper takes over).

genius Non-technical and imprecise term for a person with the highest range of mental ability and originality; sometimes refers to altogether exceptional creative achievement such as reached by Mozart in music, Shakespeare in letters, and Michaelangelo in the visual arts.

genotype The **genetic** constitution of an individual as determined by the **genes** he or she has inherited. cf. **phenotype**.

geriatric psychiatry *See* **psychiatry**.

geriatrics That branch of medicine concerned with the diagnosis, treatment and care of old people. *See also* **psychiatry, geriatric**.

gestalt Form, pattern, structure or configuration; an integrated whole which is more than a mere summation of parts. The Gestalt School of **psychology** opposed behaviourist psychology, holding that the organizational aspects of a whole entity are neglected when **behaviour** and psychological processes are studied in terms of their constituent elements.

gestalt psychology *See* **psychology**.

gestalt therapy A form of **psychotherapy** developed by Frederic Perls, who believed that **neurosis** arises out of the splitting of the 'whole' which normally unify **mind**-body and individual-environment. It focuses on awareness of current experience more than on the past or future.

gigantism Excessive height for age due to abnormal growth. Can be familial or racial, or can be due to oversecretion of growth hormone by

66

the pituitary gland during childhood. In eunuchoid gigantism the tall stature is due to delayed **puberty**, which results in continued growth of the long bones before their growing ends (epiphyses) fuse. **Epilepsy** is common, as are various mental changes.

Gilles de la Tourette syndrome Multiple **tics**, especially of the face and upper part of the body, often associated with involuntarily obscene utterances. The patient may also repeat the statements and imitate the actions of others. The condition usually has its onset in childhood and becomes chronic. The causes are unknown.

globus hystericus A sensation of a ball or globe rising from the stomach up to the throat where it produces a feeling of choking. This form of **hysterical** illness is one of the first psychiatric disorders recorded, in an Egyptian papyrus.

glue sniffing Form of solvent abuse, associated with volatile glues and cements (like model airplane cement), practised by children or adults with severe **personality** problems. The solvent may be sniffed directly from the container or soaked rag, but most commonly it is placed in a paper bag and closely applied to the nose and mouth to inhale the fumes. Plastic bags have been associated with some fatalities. The main risks are of accident during the period of acute **intoxication** which resembles **drunkenness.** Excitement and sometimes **hallucinations** occur. **Death** can happen through acute toxicity and liver necrosis.

glutethimide (Doriden) Introduced in 1954 as a safe and effective non-barbiturate **hypnotic** and widely prescribed. Its abuse potential was soon recognized. Irregular absorbtion and rapid excretion combine to produce an erratic pattern of **withdrawal symptoms,** and withdrawal **convulsions** may actually occur during continued administration.

Goldstein, Kurt (1878–1965) German neuropsychiatrist and psychologist whose pioneering studies of **aphasia** laid the groundwork for integrating psychological with anatomical factors in explaining behavioural changes associated with brain lesions.

gonadal dysgenesis *See* **dysgenesis**.

grandiosity A quality of **behaviour** and speech associated with pretentiousness, heightened self-esteem, and exaggerated ideas of personal significance, power, influence, wealth etc. Occurs as a **personality** trait and also as an element of certain illnesses, such as **hypomania** or **schizophrenia**, when it may be **delusional**.

grief Deep or intense sorrow and distress, especially following **bereavement** or other loss. May be normal, with **mourning** proceeding in appropriate stages after the death of a loved person, or pathological, when the process is distorted or prolonged (**pathological grief reaction**), or may develop into **depressive illness**.

grief reaction The normal response to the loss or **death** of a loved one. In **DSM III**, uncomplicated **bereavement**.

pathological grief reaction A **mental illness** or severe behavioural or emotional disturbance that arises as a distortion of the normal **mourning** process, often having delayed and indirect or atypical expression of sorrow with **guilt**, anger and other **symptoms** of distress.

Griesinger, Wilhelm (1817–1869) Great pioneer psychiatrist. Wrote an influential textbook *Pathologie und Therapie der psychischen Krankheiten*, 1845. Believed insanity was due to brain disorder. The first director of the university psychiatric hospital in Zurich, the Burghölzli, a post to be held much later by **Bleuler**. As professor at Berlin from 1864 he combined neurology and psychiatry.

grimacing Facial contortions often expressing pain or disgust or intended to cause amusement. In **schizophrenia**, particularly in association with other catatonic features and in some forms of **brain damage**, repeated facial contortions occur which appear to lack any communicative significance or **affective** association, and are not under the voluntary control of the subject.

Groddeck, Georg (1866–1934) Somewhat obscurantist German doctor who in *The Book of the It* (1921) described the person as influenced by unknown forces. 'I am lived by my It.' He dealt with fields later to be recognized more clearly, such as psychotherapy for patients ill with **psychoses**, and **psychosomatic disorders**.

group therapy *See* **psychotherapy, group**.

Gudden, Bernard Von German psychiatrist who studied brain degeneration. Murdered by drowning in 1886 by his patient King Ludwig II of Bavaria.

guilt Feelings of self-blame and self-reproach, and accompanying **behaviour** and utterances, which may follow realistically from infringement of a moral code or, in pathological states, which are not explicable in objective terms. If the self-blame is groundless, it may manifest as a **delusion**, common in **depressive illness**.

hair plucking   *See* **trichotillomania.**

halfway house   The term applied to a group dwelling which provides transitional accommodation between life in an institution and independent living in the community.

hallucination   Perception, e.g. auditory, visual or physical, in the absence of a corresponding external stimulus.

auditory hallucination   Subjective **perception** of voices or other sounds, in the absence of corresponding external stimuli.

hypnagogic hallucination   Visual hallucinations or vivid mental imagery experienced while falling asleep. Can occur in normal persons who are extremely fatigued; often of no pathological significance.

hypnopompic hallucinations   The apparent brief persistence of a **dream** into the waking state, making an hallucinatory experience that is fundamentally the same as a **hypnagogic** one.

lilliputian hallucination   Visual hallucinations of minute persons or objects. May be found in **organic** states particularly.

normal hallucination   Hallucinations occurring in normal individuals, e.g. on the borderline between waking and sleeping or during other alterations in the state of **conciousness; hypnagogic** hallucinations occur on wakening.

pseudo hallucination   An hallucination experience which is at least in part under voluntary control and can be called up or dispelled by an effort of will.

tactile hallucination   Sensations which are interpreted as animals, insects, electricity or foreign bodies in or under the skin. Characteristic of **cocaine psychosis.**

visual hallucination   A visual **percept** which may be simple, e.g. a flash of light, or complex, e.g. a figure or a formed object. Experienced in the absence of an external stimulus.

hallucinatory state induced by drugs   False sensory **perceptions,** occurring in the absence of stimuli, induced by a variety of **drugs** and other pharmacological agents.

hallucinogens   Substances which produce severe perceptual disturbance including **hallucinations.** The term is often used synomously with **psychedelic (mind-**altering) or **psychotomimetic** (mimicking the manifestations of **psychosis).** They include the tryptamine group **(serotonin** or **psilocybin),** the phenylethylamine group (including

hallucinosis

mescaline) and a mixed group which includes **lysergic acid diethylamide.**

hallucinosis The state of experiencing **hallucinations.**

alcoholic hallucinosis An acute or subacute disorder in **alcoholics** characterized by **hallucinations** usually of an auditory type occurring in clear **consciousness.** There is frequently a **paranoid** flavour.

chronic hallucinosis Persistent experience of **hallucinations.**

hangover 'Morning after' **syndrome** following ingestion of intoxicating quantities of alcohol, characterized by headache, photophobia, hyperacusis, bad taste, occasional nausea, vomiting and depressed **mood.** Causative factors include incomplete metabolic breakdown of alcohol and its intermediate product acetaldehyde, as well as other toxic congeners generated in the processing of the alcohol ingested.

Hartmann, H. (1884–1970) German psychoanalyst, later active in the United States.

hashish *See* **cannabis.**

hebephrenia *See* **schizophrenia, hebephrenic.**

hedonism The theory that pleasure is the greatest good. In **psychiatry** the seeking of goals because they afford gratification. The pursuit of pleasure.

Heidegger, Martin (1889–1976) German existentialist philosopher. Pupil and successor to **Husserl** as professor of philosophy at Freiburg University: 'Being-in-the-world' or **'Dasein'** was proposed as the expression of subjectivity. Ideally it is free and should be constantly striving through authentic choice and future-directed 'projects' to transcend the limits, i.e. the 'facticity' of the world. However, there are given facts which cannot be negated: we are *'thrown'* into a particular time and place ('Geworfenheit'); because we are human and part of an almost inescapable social complex, we 'forfeit' a degree of our subjective freedom to the expectations of others and the exigencies of the trivial day-to-day world. Furthermore, beyond **Dasein** is death and nothingness, and we live in constant 'dread', and are aware of the 'experience of progressing towards **death**'. Profoundly influenced **Binswanger** and the field of existential **psychiatry.**

Heller's syndrome   Disorder of infancy preceded by a few years of normal development but involving severe disturbance of **behaviour, affect,** speech and social skills. There may be overactivity and **stereotypies,** and in some cases intellectual impairment. Occasionally precipitated by overt brain disease, e.g. **encephalitis.**

hepatolenticular degeneration   Wilson's disease. A rare familial disorder of copper metabolism leading to gross **tremors,** with muscle spasticity, emotional lability and cirrhosis of the liver. Patients have greenish-brown rings at the corneo-scleral margin in the eye, due to copper deposition and known as Kayser-Fleischer rings.

hermaphrodite   A person who has sex glands containing both ovarian and testicular tissue, either as separate gonads (i.e. one ovary and one testis) or combined as an ovo-testis.

heroin   (diacetylmorphine) Made from **morphine** by the acetylation of both the phenolic and the alcoholic OH groups. Used medically in pain relief; taken by abusers initially for its euphoric effect, but later to prevent **withdrawal symptoms.** It has a high **physical dependence capacity** and is a major **drug** of **abuse** in the western world. The drug may be sniffed or subcutaneous injection is common among intermittent users, but intravenous injecting or 'shooting up' is preferred by hard-core users.

heterozygousness   (obs. heterozygosity) Relates to the **genetic** condition of a person or other organism whose two **genes** of a given factor pair are different.

hiccough   (hiccup) 1. A sudden intake of air caused by spasm of the diaphragm, followed by a closing of the glottis producing a characteristic sound. 2. A minor and transient interruption of a process. Medical name: singultus.

psychogenic hiccough   An uncommon disorder. Hiccough in response to psychological **stress** without identifiable **organic** cause.

high-grade defect   Equivalent to mild **mental retardation.**

Hippocrates (460–377 BC)   Perhaps the first layman to become a professional physician, he founded the school of Cos. Writings attributed to him formed the foundations of Western medicine and the Hippocratic oath still represents the ethical ideal of medical practice.

Hirschfeld, Magnus (1868–1935)   Writer of *Sexual Pathology*, he
founded a society to champion unfortunates with congenital handicaps in which he included **homosexuality** and other sexual variations. In 1919 he set up a marriage bureau and in 1921 organised the
First International Congress of Sexology in Paris.

homeostasis   The maintenance of constant normal internal environment in biological systems by the operation of self-regulating
processes which compensate for disruptive changes. The term is
sometimes applied, by analogy, to social systems.

homicide   The killing, whether lawful or unlawful, of one human
being by another with the exception of alien enemies killed in acts of
war. Unlawful homicide includes **murder,** manslaughter, **infanticide** and causing death by dangerous driving.

homophile organizations   Organizations of people who are concerned with the welfare and rights of homosexuals.

homosexuality   Sexuality involving people of the same sex or gender,
either as overt **behaviour** or as a sexual preference.

Horney, Karen (1885–1952)   American **psychoanalyst**, commonly
considered one of the **neo-Freudians**. Rejected **libido** theory and its
associated stages of psychosexual development. Regarded the real
self, unique to the individual, as the basis of **integration**, and the
idealized self as an essentially neurotic attribute. Resembled
Sullivan in her strong interpersonal emphasis.

hospitalism   Usually taken to refer to the effects upon young
children, from **anxiety** and irritability to gross **depression,**when
separated from parents on admission to hospital, as described by
Bowlby and the Robertsons. May be observed even during short
separations.

humoral theory   Ancient theory that health or illness was
determined by the balance of the four bodily humours, namely blood,
phlegm, yellow bile and black bile.

Huntington's chorea   A degenerative condition of the **central
nervous system** often presenting as late as the fourth and fifth
decades of life, manifested by **dementia** and progressive disorder of
movement. Small jerks of limbs, face and shoulders progress to gross
contortions of the body. The condition, eventually fatal, is transmitted by a dominant mode of inheritance, so that half the children of
the sufferer will be similarly afflicted.

Hurler's syndrome *See* **gargoylism.**

Husserl, Edmund (1859–1938)   German philosopher influential in the development of **existentialism.** Predecessor of **Martin Heidegger** at the Department of philosophy at Freiburg. He developed **phenomenology** both as a technique of analysis and an approach to the understanding of 'being' and 'existence' (ontology). The central tenet is that reality is based on the subjective experience of the factual world: 'The world is *my* world'. There is no 'being' beyond the facts of experienced time and place. Therefore to understand the experience of a particular individual, one needs to examine minutely the facts of that experience: 'back to the things themselves'.

hydrocephalus   In childhood, before the bone sutures have closed, increase in the volume of cerebrospinal fluid in the ventricles of the brain from a variety of **organic** causes, with increase in the size of the skull as well. In adulthood, increase in the intracranial pressure with headache, vomiting and drowsiness.

hyperkinesis   Extreme overactivity often of random or haphazard sort, with **distractibility.** Occurs in children, sometimes related to **brain damage** or **mental retardation.**

hyperkinetic reaction   An induced disturbance characterized by marked overactivity, **distractibility** and **short attention span.** Occurs in psychiatric illnesses such as **manic-depressive psychosis** and **schizophrenia,** and following physical illness such as **encephalitis.**

hyperkinetic syndrome   A childhood disorder in which the essential features are a grossly excessive level of activity, short **attention span** and **distractibility.** Learning is impaired. Impulsiveness, marked **mood** fluctuations and **aggression** may be associated. Developmental delay and poor interpersonal relationships are common.

hyperpnoea   Overbreathing with increased respiratory rate and excursion producing a relative carbon dioxide washout and consequent progressive respiratory alkalosis (hypocapnia). *See also* **hyperventilation.** (To be distinguished from hyperpnoea by exaggerated mental activity).

hyperpnoea, hysterical   The unconscious production of the **hyperventilation** syndrome as a **hysterical** symptom.

hypersomnia Excessive length of otherwise normal **sleep.** Most commonly it results from overdosage with **hypnotic or sedative drugs** but it can result from **encephalitis** and other brain diseases. Another cause can be psychological in origin, such as the wish to withdraw, seen frequently in depressed patients.

hyperthyroidism (syn. thyrotoxicosis) Due to excess production of thyroxine by the thyroid gland; six times as common in females, possibly precipitated by emotional crises. **Symptoms** are intolerance of heat, increased heart rate persisting when asleep, a fine **tremor,** loss of weight, protrusion of the eyes and overactivity often associated with **anxiety.**

hyperventilation Condition resulting from overbreathing due to **anxiety,** resulting in feelings of faintness, tachycardia, tingling of extremities and increased anxiety due to increased alkalosis. Dramatically reversed by breathing into a paper bag to build up the level of carbon dioxide. *See also* **carpopedal spasm; neurosis, hysterical.**

hypnobatia (obs.) The performance during **sleep** of actions that ordinarily take place when the person is awake. *See also* **somnambulism.**

hypnosis A state of heightened **suggestibility** and focused **attention** deliberately induced by a process including monotonous repetitive stimulation, accompanied by appropriate suggestions.

hypnotics **Drugs,** sedative in lower doses and producing **sleep** when given in sufficient quantity. **Barbiturates** were formerly commonly used for this purpose but have now been virtually supplanted by the **benzodiazepines.** A price is paid in that sleep is usually worse for a period when the hypnotic is withdrawn.

hypochondriasis Unrealistic interpretation of details of bodily function or physical sensations as abnormal, leading to preoccupation with the **fear** or **belief** of having a serious disease. Occurs on its own as a specific psychoneurosis or in association with other psychiatric illnesses, e.g. **neurosis, obsessional** or **schizophrenia.** *See also* **neurosis, cardiac.**

hypoglycaemia Low glucose level in the blood stream resulting in headache, mental dullness, fatigue, **confusion, hallucinations,** bizarre **behaviour,** leading to **convulsions, coma** and **death,** and as a result of increased adrenal gland activity to palpitations, **anxiety,** sweating, tremulousness and hunger. Prolonged hypoglycaemia leads to loss of cerebral function. Occurs in diabetes mellitus as a result of insulin overdosage and insufficient intake of carbohydrates. Treated by giving glucose by mouth, or injection by vein if the patient is comatose.

hypomania A mild form of **mania** though the term is often used in preference to mania, which has acquired wider colloquial usage. Patients have **mood** elevation, and are overactive and excited but **labile,** so that **euphoria** and irritability may come and go. They sleep little, but often seem physically fit and resilient. *See also* **psychosis, manic-depressive.**

hypothyroidism State of reduced thyroid function. Presents with anaemia, fatigue, lethargy, coarseness of the features of the face, dry skin, loss of hair and especially of eyebrows, gain of weight, constipation, loss of appetite, intolerance of cold. Coarse voice, mental dullness, deafness and **apathy,** occasionally **hallucinations** and **paranoid** ideas are a feature. *See also* **cretinism, myxoedema.**

hysterical Strictly, referring to **psychogenic** mechanisms of **dissociation** and **conversion** producing mainly physical symptoms. Commonly and loosely used to describe transient behavioural disturbances of dramatic attention-seeking character.

hysterical analgesia A sensory impairment which never corresponds with the cutaneous distribution of any peripheral nerve, sensory root or tract. Often occurs in a 'glove and stocking' distribution with a clear-cut upper margin.

hysterical aphonia *See* **aphonia.**

hysterical blindness Loss of vision, without physical cause, believed to result from psychological **conflict.** Pupillary responses are preserved, and the patient will blink when threatened or avoid obstacles in his path.

hysterical conversion illness A great range of bodily disorders of psychoneurotic type in which there is a transformation into physical manifestations of repressed **complexes,** or the conversion of an **emotion** into a physical **symptom.** The disturbance of function corresponds to the patient's understanding rather than to the facts of anatomy. Includes paralyses of limbs, loss or impairment of vision, deafness, numbness or sensation, disorders of gait, **tremor** etc. A mental **conflict** is dissociated and, without the patient being aware of this, obtains distorted expression in the particular symptoms. e.g. **Breuer** and **Freud's** famous case, Anna O., after nursing her father until he died, became unable to drink fluids, and by **psychotherapy** it was later discovered that she had witnessed the little dog ('horrid creature') of her lady companion drinking from a glass; recall of this repressed **memory** in an hypnotic session resulted in immediate recovery of the symptom. *See also* **dissociative state.**

hysterical epidemic Hysterical states spreading rapidly in a population by a process of sympathetic imitation, e.g. the 'dancing manias' of the Middle Ages, and as occurs in schools.

hysterical frigidity *See* **frigidity.**

hysterical fugue *See* **fugue.**

hysterical gait disturbance An abnormal gait often associated with apparent limb weakness, which is often bizarre, inconsistent and does not correspond with known neurological lesions. There are no objective neurological signs and often movement and power are normal when the patient is examined sitting or lying in bed. Occasionally a bizarre gait disturbance can be due to an extreme sensitivity to **tricyclic antidepressants,** even in small doses, especially in the elderly, and may be differentiated from the hysterical gait disturbance by measuring blood levels of the **drug,** which will usually be excessive. *See also* **astasia-abasia.**

hysterical hyperpnoea *See* **hyperpnoea** and **hyperventilation.**

hysterical mutism *See* **mutism.**

hysterical neurosis *See* **neurosis.**

hysterical pain Pain with no apparent **organic** or structural cause, which may be associated with repressed emotional **conflicts** and often has a symbolic significance. Denial of any sort of emotional conflict or psychological problem is striking in these patients.

hysterical personality disorder *See* **personality disorder.**

hysterical pseudocyesis An uncommon form of **neurosis** affecting usually a childless woman with an intense desire for pregnancy. She becomes convinced that she is pregnant and develops appropriate symptoms and signs including **amenorrhoea,** morning sickness, abdominal swelling, breast enlargement, and reports of quickening. The swelling disappears under anaesthesia and the spurious 'pregnancy' disappears with appropriate treatment, e.g. **psychotherapy.**

hysterical pseudodementia *See* **pseudodementia**

hysterical psychosis *See* **psychosis, hysterical.**

hysterical trance *See* **trance.**

hysterical tremor *See* **tremor.**

iatrogenic illness The production of harmful physical or mental changes in a patient as a result of the words, actions or prescriptions of the doctor. The most common iatrogenic illnesses are now drug-induced.

ICD-9 *Manual of the International Statistical Classification of Diseases, Injuries and Causes of Death,* Ninth Revision. (Chapter V, dealing with Mental Disorders was published separately in 1978). Geneva) World Health Organization.

id **Psychoanalytic** term devised by **Freud** *(das Es):* the part of the mind which is primal, present at birth, **unconscious,** the reservoir of psychic energy (**libido**), encompassing the instinctual **drives** of sexuality and **aggression.** Its characteristic mode is immediate, alogical pressure for satisfaction. Commonly perceived as the energetic, chaotic repository of the primitive animal part of the human **psyche.** Together with the **ego** (that part of the psyche that tests reality) and the **superego** (the conscience), it constitutes the mind. 'It is the dark, inaccessible part of our **personality** ... subject to the observance of the **pleasure principle'** (Freud). *See also* **primary process.**

idea of reference An individual's false idea that external objects or events are somehow directed towards him.

idealization A concept in psychoanalytical literature referring to overestimation of admired attributes of another person.

identification Primary identification is said to be the state of the infant when it has not yet recognized self and others as distinct. Secondary identification involves a process of adopting the **identity** of a separate other. This is the process in which the child develops an identity based on the parent, for example. The word is also used in psychoanalytical literature to refer to identification with somebody else, or seeing oneself as inside another.

identity The sense of one's continuous being as an entity distinguishable from others, providing the ability to experience oneself as having sameness, continuity and uniqueness. Identity crisis, e.g. in adolescence, refers to impairment of the sense of personal sameness and historical continuity. The sense of identity is lost in a **fugue** and can be distorted in **schizophrenia.**

identity disorder **DSM III** term signifying distress in late adolescence in which there is uncertainty over career choice, long-term goals, sexual orientation, moral values and religious affiliation.

idiocy

idiocy Historically equivalent to profound **mental retardation.**

> **amaurotic idiocy** (Tay-Sachs disease) A progressive inherited disorder of lipid metabolism, affecting the **central nervous system** with mental deterioration, progressive blindness, **epilepsy** and early **death** in cases starting in infancy. Incidence highest among Ashkenazi Jews and their descendants.

idioglossia A disturbance of speech despite normal neurological findings and adequate mental ability in which a mixture of volumes and tones is used such that the speech cannot be understood. The condition is classically seen in small children and is related to **idiolalia** and the private language of children or the mentally handicapped, which can only be grasped by close relatives. Idiophasia is similarly the use by some **schizophrenics** of an idiosyncratic language, useless for communication.

idiolalia A personal language, such as develops in some children with brain impairment resulting in word deafness.

idiot savant A child who appears to be mentally handicapped, but in one particular area such as music or mathematics appears to have outstanding ability bordering on **genius.** Sometimes considered an atypical form of **early infantile autism.**

illusion A destorted **perception** which is a misinterpretation of a real external stimulus.

> **déjà vu illusion** An intense feeling of familiarity where places, persons or events which may never have been seen before appear to be a part of the individual's past experience. Common in **temporal lobe epilepsy.**

> **jamais vu illusion** An erroneous feeling or **conviction** that familiar events, places or experiences have never happened or been seen before.

imago In **psychoanalysis** the **unconscious** mental representation or picture of an important person in the individual's life, such as a parent or those who stand for parents.

imbecile Historically equivalent to moderate **mental retardation.**

implosion *See* **flooding.**

impotence Inability to perform sexually. Usually applied to failure to achieve or maintain satisfactory erection of the penis, but is sometimes used to describe ejaculatory failure.

imprinting A tendency to show a predictable **behaviour** response to a specific stimulus which depends on exposure to the stimulus at a critical period of development. Best described in certain species of birds when selection of potential parent or sexual partner depends on such early critical exposure. Probably no direct homologue in mammalian behaviour and is of little relevance to the human.

incidence Frequency of onset of disorder. An term in **epidemiology** denoting the rate of inception of new cases per unit of population over a given period, usually expressed as annual incidence per 1000 population.

incoherence of talk A form of **thought disorder** in which the association of words and their juxtaposition as well as structure leads to meaningless speech. This is classically a sign of **schizophrenia,** but a seemingly similar condition occurs in extremes of **mania.**

incoherence of thought *See* **thought.**

incongruity of affect *See* **affect.**

incorporation A primitive **defence mechanism** by which an external object appears to be ingested or otherwise taken into the self. It can be distinguished from **introjection,** which implies that objects have been symbolically ingested.

individual psychology System of psychological theory developed by **Alfred Alder**.

infanticide Deliberate killing by a woman of her child under the age of 12 months, when the balance of her **mind** is disturbed. Occurs in numerous psychiatric disorders, including **depressive illness, sociopathy,** or in **non-accidental infancy**. The law reflects the awareness of society of post-partum risk.

infantile autism *See* **early infantile autism.**

inferiority complex *See* **complex**

inhibition 1. In **psychodynamics,** the **unconscious** restraint of instinctual impulses. 2. In **Eysenck** and in Russian psychophysiology, a low level of cerebral arousal. 3. In social terms, a shy **withdrawal** from social relationships. 4. In **central nervous system** physiology, the dampening effect of e.g. higher centres upon lower, such as the upper motor neurones on spinal reflexes.

insanity   Legal but non-psychiatric term for a severe mental illness which incapacitates a person from managing his or her own affairs. Involves responsibility for contracts, guardianship, ability to distinguish right from wrong, and necessity for commital.

insight   An awareness of the presence, significance or meaning of his **symptoms** by the patient, and their origin and role in producing his illness. This mental process may develop as a result of **psychotherapy** or through spontaneous **introspection.** Intellectual insight alone may not produce changes in **behaviour,** and emotional acceptance is often also required before meaningful or permanent changes can occur or symptoms diminish or disappear. Insight is lost in certain brain disorders and psychiatric illnesses, e.g. in **schizophrenia.**

insomnia   Sleeplessness of all kinds, i.e. inability to fall asleep, early morning waking, or sleep broken by periods of wakefulness during the night. Often a manifestation of **anxiety** or of **depressive illness.**

instinct   Originally the term was used by zoologists to describe stereotyped **drives** and **behaviour,** genetically determined, such as sucking, sexual behaviour, courting activity and species-specific activity which was necessary for survival and minimally altered by the environment. **Freud** modified the term to describe certain powerful basic drives which control our lives: the 'life' instinct and the **'death' instinct.** Not all psychoanalysts have accepted the death instinct and there is evidence that Freud himself modified his views on this in his later years. But most analysts agree that destructive drives occur in many individuals and influence behaviour adversely.

insulin therapy   (hist.) Insulin coma treatment: an obsolete form of treatment for **schizophrenia** in which **comas** were induced by insulin and relieved by oral, intragastric or intravenous glucose five or six times weekly for periods of some eight weeks. The supposed benefit is now attributed to non-specific factors associated with the treatment regime. 2. Modified insulin treatment: largely obsolete treatment intended to stimulate appetite, whereby small doses of insulin (15–20 units) are administered daily half an hour before breakfast.

integration   The process in personality development by which separate characteristics, experiences, impulses, abilities and values are gradually brought together into an organized whole. In **psychosis** a patient can be disintegrated during the illness and reintegrated on recovery. **Jung** regards integration of the self as the conscious and morally reponsible incorporation of unconscious complexes, e.g. the 'shadow', into the conscious personality.

intellect   The faculty of **mind** concerned with the **thought** processes of knowledge and **reasoning** (cognition), as opposed to the faculties of feeling **(emotion)** and will **(motivation).**

intellectualization   An **unconscious** mental **defence mechanism,** often prominent in individuals with **schizoid** or **obsessional personality disorder,** in which painful or disturbing **emotions** are displaced by **denial** of feeling and substitution of intellectual concepts and words.

intelligence   Capacity for adaptive **thought** and action, and the ability to understand and comprehend.

intelligence quotient (IQ)   An index of intellectual development, relative to the rest of the population, stated as a ratio of mental age to chronological age multiplied by 100, and thus expressed as a percentage. Most **intelligence tests** are designed so that the average IQ is 100.

intelligence test   A form of psychological test made up of a set of tasks to measure intelligence. May evaluate verbal, practical or spatial abilities, and thus consist of questions to be answered or practical tasks, e.g. block designs. *See also* **Wechsler Adult Intelligence Scale.**

interpretation   The method of clarifying and arriving at the meaning of obscure experiences of patients, such as **dreams** or **symptoms;** statements made by the clinician to the patient, attributing meanings over and above those given by the patient.

paradoxical interpretation   Approach in **psychotherapy** when the therapist invites a patient to do something, whereas in reality he wants the patient to do the opposite, and hopes that by the way he invites the patient to do this he will reject the suggestion and in fact do the contrary. Also adopted in certain **family therapy** approaches.

intersex   An anomaly of sexual differentiation when the individual's anatomical development is not completely along male or female lines, but involves some characteristics of both sexes. *See also* **hermaphrodite.**

intoxication   A state of impaired cerebral function leading to loss of **consciousness** at its most severe, generally caused by alcohol, **drug** or chemical action.

intracranial haemorrhage   Bleeding from blood vessels including arteries or veins within the skull.

intrapunitive   Of aggressive impulses that are turned on the self, in an **unconscious** assumption of **guilt** as a means of psychological defence against **anxiety** arising from interpersonal **conflict.**

introjection   A mental mechanism by which a loved or hated person can be viewed as becoming part of the individual's **personality.** This can be illustrated by the development within the child of the parental value system.

introspection   Self-observation; inward-looking examination or contemplation of the self or of one's own feelings, **thoughts, behaviour** and **motivation.** Often encouraged by **psychotherapy** and sometimes leading to **insight.**

introversion   **Behaviour** which is inward-looking, self-sufficient, solitary. The introvert **personality** shows this style habitually. (See **Jung**).

intuitive understanding   Sympathetic recognition or comprehension as a result of contemplation of reflected feelings and **insight** rather than by observation and **reasoning.** Generally applies to the understanding by one person of another's feelings, motives etc.

involutional melancholia   *See* **melancholia.**

IQ   *See* **intelligence quotient**

isolation   1. In Freudian terms, the separation of an idea from its associated emotional charge. 2. Social isolation, the separation of a person or group from wider social contacts. 3. Sensory isolation *(see* **perceptual deprivation).**

Itard, J.M.G. (1774–1838)   French educationist and hearing specialist noted for his attempts to train the 'wild boy of Aveyron'.

Jackson, John Hughlings (1835–1911)   Influential British neurologist associated with the National Hospital, Queen Square, whose lucid and prolific writings correlated disturbed **behaviour** with localized structural **brain damage.** First to describe focal lesions producing unilateral localized seizures, later called Jacksonian or focal **epilepsy.** Influenced **Freud** by his concept of hierarchical levels of brain function.

jactitation Jerking of the limbs, usually generalized and of **epileptic** origin, but occasionally a few jerks can occur with recovery from transient cerebral anoxia (e.g. a **faint**).

Jakob–Creutzfeldt disease A rapidly developing presenile **dementia** with an equal sex incidence commencing usually in the fourth or fifth decade. The early stages are marked by **anxiety,** depressed **mood,** fatigue, emotional lability, followed by impaired **memory** and concentration and an abnormal gait. In the next stage, asymmetrical neurological signs or intellectual deterioration may predominate, manifest in **delirium** with **auditory hallucinations** and **delusions,** advancing rapidly to **dementia.** The condition has been shown to be due to an organism transmissible to chimpanzees and has been accidentally transmitted from affected patients to other human subjects. It is rapidly fatal, most cases dying in less than a year. Similar in some respects to **kuru.**

jamais vu illusion *See* **illusion.**

James-Lange theory Asserts that the experience of **emotion** follows (and does not precede, as is generally assumed) the bodily changes occurring at the time of the exciting event. One is afraid because one's heart thumps, rather than that one's heart thumps because one is afraid.

James, William (1842–1910) American pragmatic philosopher and psychologist. His central concerns were the relationship of subjective experience to the external world. He enumerated three central principles: (a) 'the Will to believe', a concept of the need for action to be subjectively meaningful and ethically correct, most necessary when objective empirical facts fail unambiguously to guide a particular course of action; (b) pluralism, the right and necessity for a variety of both subjective experience and action; and (c) radical empiricism, which affirms the interaction of **thought** and the world in constant mutually adaptive relationship – the one changing the other, permitting the manipulation of the physical world as an aid to understanding. These principles underly his attempts to relate physiology and subjective **emotion**, most specifically in the **James-Lange theory** of emotion.

Janet, Pierre (1859–1947) Distinguished French student of **Charcot**, appointed by him as director of the psychological laboratory at the Salpêtrière Hospital. Best known for his concepts of **psychasthenia** which postulates a lowering of nervous or psychic tension and of **dissociation**. He accepted the hypothesis of conscious and unconscious forces in balance in the normal individual, which

Jaspers, Karl (1883–1969)

when imbalanced result in **dissociative state**. Also investigated multiple **personality**.

Jaspers, Karl (1883–1969)   Philosopher and psychiatrist, author of the famous *General Psychopathology*. He applied the principles of **phenomenology** in philosophy to problems of **neurosis** and **personality**: the psychiatrist must enter into the subjective domain of the patient's phenomenological experience of time, space, work, **emotion**, love, etc., in order to understand 'the living meaning' of the patient's existence. Furthermore, the patient is encouraged to change the apparently inescapable and fixed patterns of personality, through altered 'becoming', or **behaviour** in the world. This changed **Dasein** will reflect itself in an altered subjectivity and a change in personality. He emphasizes the patient's freedom of choice as opposed to submission to the expectation of others.

jealousy   Intense concern for the loss of affection or attention of another person, frequently accompanied by hostile feelings toward others who are perceived as rivals. It is said to be pathological if intense, and delusional if it occurs in the absence of cause. *See* **delusion**.

delusional jealousy   (syn. pathological jealousy, morbid jealousy, Othello syndrome). Jealousy of the spouse or sexual partner which not only exceeds normal bounds but in which **delusions** of infidelity are formed. Everyday events are interpreted as confirming the suspected sexual liaison and pleas for confession if acceded to are often followed by violence.

Jellinek, Elvin Horton (1890–1963)   An authority on **alcholism** research who was an exponent of the disease concept of alcoholism. Director of the Yale School of Alcohol Studies until 1950.

judgement   The mental process of discernment by **reasoning** and intuition, combining information of several kinds to reach a balanced viewpoint or decision.

Jung, Carl Gustav (1875–1961)   Swiss psychoanalyst and early associate of **Freud**. Later developed his own school of **psychoanalysis, Analytical Psychology**. He differed profoundly from Freud in his conception of the **unconscious** and the nature of the **libido**. He conceived of the unconscious as the '**collective unconscious**' and the '**personal unconscious**'. The 'collective unconcious' is a 'transpersonal' entity common to all human beings, containing a number of prefiguring dispositions. The individual through the individuation of his own life constructs his **personal identity.** Archetypes are expressed in the universal imagery of **dreams,** myths and art: the mother, child, father, wise woman, the hero, etc. Parts of the unconscious may split off to become 'splintered personalities' giving rise to **complexes**, e.g. 'the maternal complex'. Other 'archetypal' configurations include the **persona**, the mask presented to the world, i.e. the social self, such as the 'doctor' or the 'actor'. The **shadow** is the negative repressed part of the individual projected onto others in symbolic dreams. The animus is the woman's undeveloped masculinity, and the anima the man's undeveloped feminity. The personal unconscious is individual and specific and contains repressed material which was at one time conscious. Jung conceived of the **libido** as the energy underlying all psychic activity, dreams, **fantasies**, art, as opposed to Freud's conception of an essentially erotic libido. Jung separated individuals into two personality types: the externally sensitive extrovert who directs energy outward, and the introvert whose energies and sensitivity are inwardly directed.

The goal of **psychotherapy** is to permit the individual to become what he essentially is: to encourage 'individuation'. During this process the archetypes and complexes which are to varying degrees in conflict with the **ego**, are brought into consciousness through the examination of the symbolic content of dreams, fantasies and other communications. **Dreams** are given great value, for they are thought to express not only the present state of the patient, but are also 'prophetic', and may guide the patient's future **behaviour**.

Kahlbaum, Karl Ludwig (1828–1899) German psychiatrist concerned with the identification and description of distinct illnesses which he called 'symptom complexes'. A pioneer of **descriptive psychiatry**.

Kallmann, F.J. (1897–1965) German-born psychiatrist who did pioneering research in the genetic theory of **schizophrenia** at the New York Psychiatric Institute through an ingenious design studying identical and non-identical twins and their families. He showed that the risk of schizophrenia was greatest in monozygotic twins and less in dizygotic twins, even when raised apart. Established clinics for **genetic counselling**.

Kanner, Leo (1894–1981) Father of child psychiatry. Born in Austria, he received his M.D. at Berlin. In 1924 emigrated to South Dakota. Wrote on syphulis in North American Indians, and studied with **Meyer** at the Johns Hopkins Hospital, Baltimore. Published *Child Psychiatry* in 1935. Described **early infantile autism** (**Kanner's syndrome**) in 1943.

Kanner's syndrome

Kanner's syndrome   The form of **childhood psychosis** first described by distinguished American child psychiatrist Leo **Kanner** and
equivalent to **early infantile autism.** Does not include other
childhood psychoses nor autistic children with organic brain
impairments.

Kierkegaard, Søren (1813–1855)   Danish philosopher, generally
regarded as the originator of **existentialism**. A theologian, he based
much of his writing on the events of his personal life, notably his
agonizing over giving up his fiancée Regina, and his crises of
religious faith. He believed subjective experience was the only guide
to truth. Faith in objective standards and meaning, particularly
Christianity, was absurd. In the face of this absurdity **belief** requires
a 'leap of faith', based on personal **conviction**, and moral beliefs; and
acting according to objective expectations of religion or society is an
act of 'bad faith', and is 'inauthentic', as opposed to an 'authentic'
existence derived from choice based on inner conviction. The lack of
external guidance and validation undermines certainty and inner
peace and generates constant **anxiety** or angst, and we pass our lives
in 'fear and trembling'.

Kinsey, Alfred Charles (1894–1956)   A zoologist and student of
human sexual **behaviour**, Director of the Institute of Sex Research
at Indiana University. *Sexual Behaviour in the Human Male* was
published in 1948 and the corresponding volume on *Female Sexuality*
in 1953. These volumes were based upon 18 500 personal interviews
and demonstrated the wide variations in human sexual behaviour.
Although these studies have been strongly criticized on method-
ological grounds they remain important milestones in the study of
human sexuality.

Kinsey scale   A graded scale introduced by **Kinsey** and his colleagues
to describe the range of variation in heterosexual and homosexual
behaviour. A Kinsey rating of 0 means exclusively heterosexual, 6
exclusively homosexual and 3 equal involvement in hetero- and
homosexuality. Scale normally applied to a defined period of time
(e.g. during the past 3 years).

Klein, Melanie (1882–1960)   Child therapist, generally regarded as
the founder of the British school of **psychoanalysis**. She placed great
emphasis on psychic development in early infancy. The infant's
psychic life is dominated by the process of introjecting objects and
there is a constant struggle to retain and incorporate good objects and
project the bad objects. Aggressive drives dominate the first two years
of life, and a primitive **superego** is formed during the first year.
Furthermore, the infant is held to be aware of the parents' sexual

activity and in her view the **Oedipus complex** is formed during the first few months of life, and is derived from the infant's wish to penetrate, destroy and incorporate the mother's body which in turn contains the father's penis. These aggressive impulses generate a fear of retaliation, and a 'paranoid position' towards the world dominates the first year of psychic development. During this period the mother is experienced as a fragmented collection of good and bad parts. With the later realization that the mother is a unitary figure, with both good and bad aspects, **guilt** develops because of the destructive **fantasies** which have been directed at the incorporated good aspects of the mother and the **'depressive position'** develops. It becomes the basis of the capacity for love. Klein analysed very young children and characteristically gave direct interpretations on the basis of their play, conversation, etc. The primary focus is the analysis of **object relations**, with the goal of developing a realistic response to the sadistic impulses, and the capacity to identify with real and introjected good objects.

kleptomania   A condition in which the patient has an inner **compulsion** to take things, for which he often has no use. He is unable to resist the urge to steal.

Klinefelter's syndrome   An abnormality of the sex **chromosomes** when there is an extra X chromosome (XXY), resulting in a **syndrome** of tall, sterile males with a tendency towards feminine body fat distribution.

koro   A particular form of **anxiety** illness occurring in South-East Asia associated with a **belief** that the penis will retract into the abdomen and death will result.

Korsakoff, Sergei S. (1853–1900)   Russian neurologist. *See also* **Korsakoff psychosis, Wernicke's syndrome**.

Kraepelin, Emil (1856–1926)   Great German psychiatrist, professor at Heidelberg and then Munich, who described **dementia praecox** and **manic-depressive** insanity, and was regarded as the father of **descriptive psychiatry**. Contemporary psychiatry, as far as **signs**, **symptoms** and **syndromes** are concerned, still rest on the major subdivisions between disorders set out in his famous textbook of 1883, on the basis of the natural history (onset and course) of mental disorders as well as their form of presentation.

Krafft-Ebing, Richard von (1840–1903)   Neuropsychiatrist and early student of sexual pathology, Professor of Psychiatry in Strasburg, his interests ranged through insanity, **sexual deviation**,

Kretschmer Ernst (1888–1964)

epilepsy, paralysis agitans and hemicrania. He established the relationship between syphilis and general paralysis of the insane; now remembered for his *Psychopathia Sexualis*, a pioneering study of sexual aberrations published in 1886.

Kretschmer Ernst (1888–1964) German psychiatrist who advanced views on the importance of **physique** in mental illness.

kuru A subacute degenerative brain disorder leading to **dementia,** limited to the Fore tribe in New Guinea. A transmissible infective organism, possibly a virus may be involved.

labile mood *See* **mood.**

Laing, Ronald D. (1927–) Scottish psychiatrist, **psychoanalyst** and antipsychiatrist. Widely read radical critic of psychiatric treatments and attitudes towards **schizophrenia.** Asserted schizophrenic symptoms to be understood as **adaptation** and defence against a threatening and ambiguous personal environment. The family of the schizophrenic, rather than the patient, is a pathological nexus of mutually inter-dependent and mutually destructive individuals. Practising psychiatrists and psychiatric institutions are regarded as instruments of society, and their therapies Laing labelled 'degradation ceremonies'. More recently, interested in the influence of intra-uterine experiences on later development.

lalling Very severe **stammering** which makes speech almost impossible to understand.

lanugo hair A fine downy hair found, particularly on the face and back, in patients with severe **anorexia nervosa** and other debilitating conditions. Also fine hair covering the fetus and shed in the seventh month of gestation.

lapsus linguae *See* **parapraxis.**

latah A form of **hysterical** illness occurring especially, though not exclusively, in South-East Asia. Extreme **suggestibility, automatic obedience, echolalia** and **echopraxia** are among the characteristic features.

latency stage In **psychoanalysis,** the period of **personality development** between the age of 5 (end of **Oedipal stage**) and **puberty** when sexual **drive** and activity are postulated to be dormant. The child during this stage is preoccupied to learn and gain skills ('tutor-prone'). It is now apparent through observation and research that sexual thoughts and activity do indeed occur in many children during this time.

latent content In **psychoanalysis,** the hidden meaning or significance of a **thought,** feeling, action, **symptom** or other mental experience. Of a **dream,** its meaning as revealed by the associations to its content made by the dreamer when awake, assisted by the **interpretations** of the therapist. cf. **manifest content.**

Laurence-Moon-Biedl syndrome (syn. retinodiencephalic degeneration) Degeneration of the retina with **obesity, mental retardation** and genital abnormality occurring in families.

learning Any change in **behaviour** that results from experience. Ordinary learning can occur from imitation, or from trial-and-error, or as a result of teaching or of training in the case of complex skills.

learning disability 1. Specific: retardation in the acquisition of one or more educational skills, as compared with a child's expected level of functioning on the basis of age and general level of **intelligence.** 2. General: disability associated with low **intelligence quotient.**

learning theory A large body of concepts to do with the process of learning, including **associationism** and the various other theories of **cognition** and **conditioning.** No one theory of learning has gained general acceptance.

left-handedness A state in which preference is given to the left hand for skilled actions; by itself a normal variation. Some view educational influences to convert preferred motor activity to right-handedness as a cause of **learning** difficulties. Either the right hemisphere of the brain is dominant in left-handedness, or neither hemisphere has a clear dominance. If undisturbed motor activity is allowed to develop, of no clinical significance.

lesbian A female with **homosexual** preferences in sexual attraction and **behaviour.**

lesbianism **Homosexuality** involving members of the female sex.

leucotomy A psychosurgical operation to destroy neural connections with or remove part of the prefrontal areas of the brain's frontal lobes, aimed to reduce severe tension, in patients suffering from **obsessional neurosis,** chronic **anxiety** illness schizophrenia etc. Can lead to **apathy** and irresponsibility; hence it is adopted rarely and when other treatments have failed.

Lewin, Kurt (1890–1947) German-American social psychologist. Held academic posts at Cornell University and Massachussetts Institute of Technology where he was Director of the Research Center for Group Dynamics at the time of his death. Notable for his application of field theory to psychology. He defined the field as 'the totality of coexisting facts which are conceived of as mutually interdependent'. He proposed that to grasp an individual's **behaviour**, it was necessary to understand the total contextual field in which he existed at a particular moment. The combination of the individual and the field constituted the psychological 'life space'. Influenced the theory of group **psychotherapy**.

Lewis, Aubrey (1900–1975) Distinguished Australian-born British psychiatrist who joined the staff of the Maudsley Hospital in 1928 and became Clinical Director of its Institute of Psychiatry in 1936. Appointed Professor of Psychiatry, University of London in 1945, knighted in 1959. Under his leadership the Maudsley Hospital, combined with the Bethlem Royal Hospital in 1948, became a world centre of psychiatric teaching and research.

libido Used loosely to describe sexual drive or interest. A **psychoanalytic** term for emotional energy which is sexual in nature.

limbic system A network of neurones passing through the amygdala, hippocampus and mammilliary bodies at the base of the brain, thought to be intimately concerned with **memory** and emotional function.

lipochondrodystrophy *See* **gargoylism.**

lisping A disorder of articulation in which hissing sounds (sibilants) are replaced or mispronounced, usually due to incorrect placing of the tongue in relation to the upper teeth. Sometimes this is a **functional** mannerism, and a sign of immaturity, but in some patients it is a problem requiring orthodontic treatment.

lithium A naturally occurring element in the same category as sodium and potassium, which it can displace and vice versa. Was used for many years to treat various ailments such as gout and kidney disease, but in the last decade has been found useful in the treatment of the **affective disorders,** particularly in the prevention of **mania.** It is less effective than the **phenothiazines** in the management of acute mania. Periodic tests of the serum level are required to monitor the continuous use which is necessary, as it can be toxic or even fatal. Signs of toxicity include unstable gait, **tremor** of the limbs, diarrhoea and mental **confusion.**

lobotomy *See* leucotomy; psychosurgery.

lobotomy syndrome Undesirable sequelae of **psychosurgery** (prefrontal **leucotomy**) including states of **apathy,** irresponsibility or disinhibition.

logorrhoea An almost interminable outpouring of words, sometimes seen in **mania** and **schizophrenia,** and in the presence of **brain damage.**

Lombroso, Cesare (1836–1909) Italian psychiatrist interested in criminology. He regarded criminals as a sort of surviving primitive race, akin to the earlier notion about 'degeneration' of the French clinicians **Morel** and **Moreau.**

love object A **psychoanalytic** term for a person or thing outside the self to which **libido** is directed.

LSD *See* lysergic acid diethylamide.

lunacy An out-dated term for a mental disorder which qualified the sufferer to be committed to an **asylum.**

lunatic An out-dated term for a mentally disordered individual who was liable to confinement in an **asylum.**

Luria, Alexander Romanovich (1902–1977) Russian neuropsychologist who studied speech deficits in aphasia, relating the neurological impairments to psychological mechanisms and effects. He developed the treatment of **aphasia,** combining physical and psychological techniques for victims of brain trauma.

lying Occurs as a form of antisocial behaviour in some disturbed children, sometimes together with truancy and stealing. *See also* **pathological lying**. Often a defensive manoeuvre to maintain self-esteem in the face of external catastrophe or personal failings.

lysergic acid diethylamide (LSD) (sl. 'acid') A **psychedelic** drug originally derived from ergot but now available synthetically, which produces when ingested orally in minute doses (micrograms) marked perceptual changes, usually **visual hallucinations, synaesthesias** and **mood** changes in the presence of a clear **sensorium**. The effects are different from **schizophrenia** in which **auditory hallucinations** predominate, so the earlier hope that the LSD response could be a model of, and thus a basis for study of schizophrenia has proved untrue.

macropsia   Visual experience when things appear larger than they should in relation to other sensory cues. It can occur transitorily as part of an epileptic **aura** or **migraine,** but lesions anywhere in the visual system from retina to brain cortex can cause it. *See also* **micropsia.**

maladjustment   Impaired ability to behave and relate to others in a way that fosters the person's own concerns and interests, and gives appropriate consideration to the well-being of others.

malaria therapy   A major advance in the treatment of cerebral syphilis introduced by Wagner Von Jauregg in 1917. The patient was infected with benign tertian malaria and after ten or more rigors the condition was aborted with quinine. In most cases the recurrent fever was sufficent to destroy the heat-sensitive spirochaete causing the syphilis. Later replaced by 'heat box' treatment then rendered unnecessary by penicillin.

malingering   The simulation of **symptoms** of illness or injury with intent to deceive. Common in cases where criminal prosecution, personal injury, compensation or military service are involved. The overlap with **hysterical** reactions is often dependent upon the degree to which **motivation** for the deception is conscious or **unconscious.** *See also* **factitious disorder, Munchausen syndrome; neurosis, compensation.**

mania   1. *See* **manic illness.** 2. (obs.) Denotes a morbid impulse or exaggerated feeling for behaving in a forbidden or harmful way (such as **kleptomania** or compulsive stealing, **pyromania** or fire-setting, **erotomania** or delusional **belief** by a woman that a man is deeply in love with her, etc.)

manic   Manifesting violent or unrestrained **behaviour** when in the manic phase of a **manic-depressive illness.**

manic illness   One of the two major forms of **manic-depressive illness;** a **psychosis** characterized by excessive elation of **mood,** increased activity amounting to restlessness, rapid **thought** and speech to the point of incoherence **(flight of ideas). Judgement** is impaired so that the patient endangers his own interests. **Behaviour** is distorted by undue self-importance, sometimes amounting to **delusions** of grandeur. Treatment is with **drugs** such as **pheno-thiazines** or **lithium.** Hospital admission is usually necessary to deter the patient from acting against his own interests (by impulsive mistakes, extravagance, or overbearing behaviour to others which is at times aggressive).

manic type   One form of **manic-depressive psychosis.**

manic-depressive   Of an illness or an individual who suffers from the **psychosis** which has both manic and depressive phases.

manic-depressive illness   The most distinct form of the **affective disorders,** manifesting in **depressive illness** or **manic illness,** either occurring in phases. Some patients have both at different times (bipolar) or only recurrent depressive illness (unipolar). This term is to be preferred to **psychosis,** since some patients with abnormal **mood** disorder may maintain adequate contact with reality. *See also* **psychosis, manic-depressive.**

manifest content   In **psychoanalysis,** the **dream** as reported by the dreamer. cf. **latent contact.**

mannerism   Idiosyncratic motor **behaviour** which tends to be repetitive and seems pointless, e.g. a gesture. Occurs in **schizophrenia** and may have symbolic significance.

manneristic   *See* **mannerism;** *see also* **echo reactions.**

MAOI   Drugs *See* **monoamine oxidase inhibitors.**

maple syrup urine disease   A brain impairment, caused genetically but manifesting after birth, associated with defective decarboxylation of branch-chained keto acids, which gives the urine a smell like that of maple syrup. Death at the age of about two years is frequent. There is usually profound **mental retardation** and defective motor development in those who survive untreated. Treatment consists of a diet low in branch-chained amino acids. Originally described as Hartnup disease.

marijuana   *See* **cannabis.**

marital disharmony   Failure of accord and reciprocity between the two partners in a marriage, mutual distrust being expressed as discordant feelings and actions.

marital infidelity   Failure of trust and loyalty by one or both partners in a marriage, especially as expressed by lack of sexual faithfulness; it can be imagined about a spouse, as in delusional **jealousy.**

marital problems   A difficulty within a marriage, reflecting some aspect of the relationship between the partners which is affected by

behavioural, temperamental or sexual incongruities or incom-
patibilities.

marriage guidance   Assistance to a married couple by a trained lay
counsellor belonging to the Marriage Guidance Council, aiming to
clarify and resolve problems in their relationship, usually in a series
of meetings.

masochism   Sexual gratification that results from experiencing pain
or humiliation. Closely related to **sadism** and to **bondage.**
Sometimes used in a more general sense when self-inflicted discomfort or humiliation is apparently rewarding.

masturbation   The act of physically stimulating the penis or clitoris,
most often with the hand, for sexual pleasure and, usually, **orgasm.**
Commonly, erotic thoughts or images accompany the physical stimulation (masturbation **fantasy).**

maternal overprotection   Over-indulgence and pampering in
childhood, so that self-reliance and tolerance of disappointment are
not learned; a predisposing factor leading to later limitations of
personality or **neurosis.**

maternal rejection   Instead of affection and succour, dislike and
withdrawal by the parent from a child. Can occur with psychiatric
illness or **personality disorder** of the mother, and can predispose a
child to later psychiatric illness or difficulties in relationships with
others.

Maudsley, Henry (1835–1918)   British psychiatrist, after whom
the famous hospital in London is named, who believed that mental
phenomena arose from the physical structure of the brain and that
behavioural aberrations could be explained on the basis of defects in
this structure. He eschewed metaphysics as anathema.

Mayer-Gross, Willi (1889–1961)   German psychiatrist who came to
Britain in the 1930s and became an important educative influence in
bringing Continental psychiatry and **phenomenology** to the British
scene.

McNaughton rules   A set of rules established by eleven judges in
1843, in response to a request from the House of Lords, for
determining the circumstances in which insanity may exempt an
individual from legal **responsibility** for a criminal act. The request
by the House of Lords followed the acquittal on the ground of insanity
of Daniel McNaughton on a charge of murdering William Drum-
mond, Private Secretary to Sir Robert Peel, the Prime Minister.

medical model   An approach to **mental illness** and behavioural abnormality emphasizing medical skills and knowledge as the proper basis for the work of the **psychiatrist.** It relates to a set of expectations regarding the doctor-patient relationship, including diagnosis, outcome, treatment and responsibility for patient care. This approach is contrasted with the **psychodynamic** approach. Models are useful as illustrations or examples of patterns of **behaviour,** but can be counter-productive when used as the basis for uncritical generalization, whether laudatory or derogatory.

meditation   Eastern practice adapted to western needs in which the subject engages in deep contemplation of the self, spiritual matters or other universals, and loses awareness of worldly cares. Achieved by a variety of learned techniques, sometimes involving mental excercises in silent groups; accompanied by physiological changes, and reported to be effective in relieving tension and **anxiety.**

Meduna, Ladislas J. von (1896–1964)   Hungarian born American psychiatrist who induced convulsions intended to be therapeutic first by camphor and then by cardiazol given by vein, a method now replaced by **electroconvulsive therapy.**

megalomania   Grandiose ideas of self-importance that may occur in various psychiatric illnesses such as **mania, general paresis** and **schizophrenia.**

melancholia (arch.)   A severe **depressive illness** with **symptoms** of biological dysfunction and **delusions of guilt.**

involutional melancholia   Depressive **psychosis** occurring in middle life with marked **agitation** and **delusions** (e.g. of sin and **guilt),** in people with no previous **mental illness.**

memory   A general term referring to the power of storing past experiences and of recalling them into **consciousness** with the realization that their recollection is a retrieval. Also used to refer to a specific element of experience recalled. Memory is a process, not simple storage, of **engrams,** for example, and there is some evidence of different mechanisms in short-term (seconds) and long-term memorization. Because of memory a person has a life history which is construed as a central aspect of the self. *See also* **learning; remembering.**

screen memory   **Psychoanalytic** term referring to an emotion-laden memory recalled as an apparent 'explanation' of a **symptom** or of disturbed **behaviour;** but this memory in itself, though probably

memory disturbance

real, is a cover-up or **denial** of a more traumatic and usually earlier experience repressed and recoverable only by the usual **free association** techniques, and it is the origin (in part at least) of the symptom.

memory disturbance   Any disorder of the **memory** functions whether of **registration,** retention, **recall** or recognition. The disorders are varied in character and in cause.

meningitis   Inflammation of membranes covering the brain and the spinal cord.

menopausal disorder   Psychiatric illness occurring in the female at the time of the **menopause.**

menopause   The cessation of menstruation and hence the ability to conceive and have children. Occurs between thirty years of age and the late fifties. **Symptoms** are hot flushes, palpitations and dryness of the mucous membrane lining the vagina. Related to a change in balance of the sex hormones in the body. *See also* **climacteric.**

mens rea   The requisite blameworthy state of **mind** that must be proven to exist in an individual in order for him to be convicted of certain **crimes**, such as malice or negligence.

mental age   The mean age of children in the population whose mental abilites are at the level of the child in question.

mental clouding   The impairment of **consciousness** which is found in **organic confusional states** when **attention** can be focused for short periods only.

mental deficiency   *See* **mental retardation.**

Mental Health Acts   The Acts of Parliament governing the care of the mentally ill and disordered in Great Britain, most recently 1983 (England) and 1984 (Scotland).

Mental Health Act Commission   This body is concerned with the care and welfare of individual detained patients in England and Wales, monitors the operation of the Mental Health Act 1983 and is required to visit all mental hospitals regularly. It consists of members appointed from the Law, nursing, psychology, social work, and medicine; the medical members also have a role in pronouncing on questions of treatment administered to the compulsorily detained.

Mental Health Review Tribunal These tribunals consist of three members, one legal one medical, and one lay, and were set up by the Mental Health Act 1959 to hear appeals by patients or the relatives against a patient's detention. The tribunals were given investigative powers and can order the patient's discharge, or a change in his status.

mental illness A lay term applied to the whole range of psychiatric disorders. Legally it describes one of the categories of persons to whom the **Mental Health Acts** may apply.

mental mechanism *See* **defence mechanism**

mental retardation (syn. mental deficiency, mental handicap, mental subnormality) Intellectual handicap below the statistically normal range of variation in **intelligence quotient**. Mild, moderate, severe and profound refer to four degrees that were arbitrarily defined on **intelligence tests** as being between 70 and 50, 49 and 35, 34 and 21 and below 20, respectively. Nowadays social criteria are also included in the subgrouping, reintroducing concepts similar to those originally differentiating idiots, **imbeciles** and the feeble-minded. For example, the lowest grade are unable to guard themselves from common dangers, the middle group can perform routine tasks under supervision but cannot support themselves, and the mild can contribute considerably to their own living in sheltered circumstances such as local authority homes, or hospitals, or with care-givers such as parents. Oligophrenia is a synonym (=small mindedness) derived from Greek and now little used.

mental subnormality *See* **mental retardation.**

Mental Welfare Commission for Scotland A body set up in 1960 'generally to exercise protective functions in respect of persons who may, by reason of mental disorder, be incapable of adequately protecting their persons or their interests'. This body has the power of a court of law to compel evidence, monitors the operation of powers of detention, may order the discharge of detained patients, and is required to visit Scottish mental hospitals, providing an annual report to Parliament. It also has important functions with regard to detained patients who are required to take treatment against their will. (Mental Health [Scotland] Acts 1960 and 1984.)

meperidine (pethidine) A synthetic **analgesic drug** which can cause **dependence**, originally studied as an atropine-like agent, which despite its chemical lack of similarity with **morphine** is a powerful

meprobamate

and widely used **narcotic** analgesic. Since intravenous use increases the incidence and severity of untoward effects and subcutaneous injection causes considerable local irritation, the drug is usually administered orally or by intramuscular injection.

meprobamate (Equanil; Miltown) A carbamic acid ester of glycol which has been widely used as a **tranquillizer** or **anxiolytic** agent. There are serious doubts regarding its effectiveness as a **sedative,** but it can produce both physical and psychological **dependence.**

Merleau-Ponty, Maurice (1908–1961) French philosopher whose major book *Phenomenology of Perception* was published in 1945. Professor of Psychology at the Sorbonne, he wrote extensively about the relation a person has to his own body, observing that this object is the only object around which it is not even in principle possible to take a stroll, the only object one cannot take one's leave of or turn one's back upon. He also wrote on Marxism, language, literature and the arts.

mescaline A naturally occurring **psychedelic** compound found in the peyote cactus, less potent than **lysergic acid diethylamide,** but capable of producing the same perceptual distortions and effects on **mood.**

Mesmer, Franz Anton (1734–1815) A flamboyant Viennese physician who gave his name to **mesmerism.** He believed that his theory of **animal magnetism** was a scientific and logical explanation of the phenomena which were the foundation of his fame. Although somewhat discredited as a serious figure in the history of **psychology**, he deserves his place as a founder of modern **hypnosis**, and in the early history of dynamic psychiatry and **psychotherapy.**

mesmerism (syn. **hypnosis**) The method based on the ideas of **Mesmer.** The phenomena induced in subjects were attributed to **animal magnetism.**

mesomorph A term describing a type of body build or somatotype identified by Sheldon and corresponding to **Kretschmer's** athletic type, characterized by muscular physique. Mesomorphs are said to suffer from an excess of **manic-depressive illness.** See **ectomorph, endomorph, typology.**

methadone (Physeptone) A synthetic **narcotic analgesic** which has a chemical structure only remotely resembling **morphine** but pharmacological properties qualitatively similar to those of the natural alkaloid. It is effective orally and its relatively slow onset and protracted duration of action led to its widespread use in the 'treatment' of **heroin dependence.** Although the dependence potential is less than that of morphine, methadone is none the less a **drug** of **addiction.**

methaqualone (Quaalude) A 2,3-disubstituted quinazolone introduced in 1965 as a non-**barbiturate,** non-addictive **sedative.** Soon in widespread use in medical practice, it was also a popular street drug in multi-drug abuse. In combination with diphenhydramine (Mandrax) it was found to cause **convulsions** and cerebral irritability in overdose. Alone or in combination it is associated with physical and psychological **dependence.**

Meyer, Adolf (1866–1950) Swiss neuropathologist who emigrated to the United States and became the leading figure in American **psychiatry** during the first half of the 20th Century. He served at the Worcester State Hospital in Massachusetts, and at the New York State Psychiatric Institute where he organized the first psychiatric outpatient clinic in New York City. In 1909 became Professor of Psychiatry at Johns Hopkins University, Baltimore, an important centre for the training of psychiatrists. He developed a classification of patients according to a system of reaction types. His theory of **'psychobiology'** emphasized the importance of biographical study in understanding the **personality.** His contributions to psychiatry also included emphasis on the interactive nature of **symptoms** and the unity of biological, psychological, and social functioning.

Meynert, Theodore (1833–1892) Viennese neuroanatomist, neuropathologist and neurologist, who believed that each stimulus which entered the central nervous system reached a specific area in the brain. He proposed that mental disorders could be classified according to the location of disturbances in brain functioning. According to his theory, **psychoses** result from changes in blood flow within the brain. Meynert was Director of the Psychiatric Institute in Vienna where **Freud** received training in neurology, neuropathology and psychiatry.

microcephaly Congenital defect in brain development leading to abnormally small brain and skull formation.

micropsia Things appearing smaller than they should in relation to other sensory cues. It can occur transitorily as part of an **epileptic aura** or **migraine prodrome,** but lesions anywhere in the visual system from retina to brain cortex can cause it. *See also* **macropsia.**

migraine The common form is a throbbing unilateral headache, often with nausea, vomiting and other **autonomic nervous system** symptoms and preceded by a **prodrome,** usually of a special sense experience (most typically scotomata, or flashes of light known as **fortification spectra).** The **symptoms** are probably due to cerebral spasm of blood vessels in the brain, of unknown cause but probably in most cases precipitated by hypersensitivity to circulating cate-cholamines that may be produced by certain foods in some sufferers. The clinical picture is often extended to a wide variety of repetitive stereotyped attacks of pain, even in areas other than the head, e.g. abdominal migraine. Most sufferers are aware that psychological stresses often predispose to attacks.

milieu therapy Type of therapy in which the environment, surround-ings or social setting, particularly in its emotional aspects, is deliberately used as a major element in the therapeutic process. The movement based on this theoretical approach has transformed psychiatric hospitals.

mind (syn. **psyche**) Abstract noun which denotes the totality of mental processes in the individual human being which are experi-enced or expressed as **perceptions, thoughts,** wishes, desires, feelings, acts of the will, and **behaviour,** and the organization of these events and processes.

mongolism *See* **Down's syndrome.**

Moniz, Egas (1874–1955) Portugese neurologist who introduced the operation of **leucotomy** first performed in 1935 by his surgical associate Almeida Lima. His other major contribution was cerebral angiography. Received the Nobel prize for medicine in 1949.

monoamine oxidase inhibitors (MAOI) A type of **antidepres-sant drug** less often prescribed because of toxicity and side effects in current practice than the **tricyclic antidepressants** and used for phobic states, and treatment-resistant and atypical **depressive illness.** These drugs act both inside and outside the brain to produce an irreversible inhibition of cytoplasmic monoamine oxidase. Ingest-ing foods rich in tyramine (cheese, chianti-like wines, broad beans, liver, pickled herring and chocolate) may result in severe paradoxical hypertension, cerebral bleeding, headache and stroke. **Death** has been known to occur. **Sedatives** or pethidine in combination may also result in adverse reactions.

monopolar With reference to **depressive illness,** refers to a gen-etically distinct form of the illness in which recurrent episodes of depression occur without **manic** episodes.

mood The **affective** state of a person. The term usually refers to the longer-lasting state of the patient (days or weeks) rather than to the reactive momentary changes evoked by **stress** or stimuli.

labile mood refers to frequent (hours or minutes) changes and may be regarded as abnormal only by arbitrary standards.

delusional mood A subjective sense of tense uneasiness or **perplexity** in which the individual knows that something is going on around him, directly related to himself, but he does not know what it is. From this state **delusions** (ideas or **perceptions**) may crystallize and for the patient seemingly render his previous state understandable.

Moreau de Tours, Jacques (1804–1884) French psychiatrist propounding with **Morel** the **degeneration** theory, and believing that the same hereditary predisposition affected both the insane and criminals. At the same time he influenced interest in **dynamic** psychiatry of such successors as **Janet**. *See also* **Lombroso**.

Morel, Benedict Augustin (1809–1873) French psychiatrist who proposed the **degeneration theory** of psychiatric disorders, which he regarded as deviations from the normal human state and transmissable by heredity. The first members of a degenerate family might be no more than nervous, the second generation neurotic, the third psychotic, and the fourth idiots who would die out. The **degeneration theory** dominated French psychiatry for several decades. *See also* **Lombroso**.

Moreno, J. L. (1890–1974) Austrian psychiatrist who introduced **psychodrama** and helped develop **group therapy**. He devised the method of sociometry, by which relations people have with others can be charted. Working latterly in the United States.

Morita therapy A therapy based on **Zen** Buddhism in which strict internal and external discipline, intensive work and repeated denial of **symptoms** and illness together with a frank examination of the self enable the patient to live in the community without complaint. The therapy was developed by Dr Shoma Morita who found it appealed to his Japanese patients suffering from **neurotic** or **personality disorders**.

moron Equivalent to mild **mental retardation** but often applied colloquially to all persons with mental handicap.

morphine

morphine The most important phenanthrene alkaloid of opium to which it gives its predominant pharmacological characteristics; these are the **narcotic** action manifested by analgesia, drowsiness, **mood** change and **mental clouding** together with nausea, vomiting, gastrointestinal effects and respiratory depression in larger doses. Because of the later effects most **opiate** abusers prefer diacetylmorphine or other synthetic opiates.

motivation The process which arouses, sustains, directs and regulates activity; the **drives,** goals and needs of an individual leading him to undertake particular actions. In a behaviourist approach motivation is provided by offering incentives and rewards. Classically, one of the three areas of **mind,** the others being the will **(volition)** and **emotion (affect).**

mourning Normal **grief,** the response to the death of a loved person in contrast to **depressive illness, melancholia,** or pathological **grief reaction.** Mourning enables the individual to come to terms with the loss; the time-limited process follows a predictable path with psychological and physical symptoms clearly resembling melancholia, but in which there is a preoccupation with the image and memories of the deceased.

Munchausen syndrome Persistent repetitive attendance at hospitals and clinics demanding treatment for simulated medical or surgical emergencies. **Antisocial personality** features are common. The condition is more common in males than in females. In **DSM-III,** classified as a **factitious disorder**.

murder Unlawful killing with malice aforethought.

mutism A state of not speaking, the apparent dumbness occurring although the speech mechanism is intact. Often due to **fear** of a person or situation, e.g. in a child being admitted to hospital. It is frequently seen in **schizophrenia,** especially **catatonia,** and in severe **depressive illness.** Elective mutism can occur when the patients speaks only in particular situations or to certain people.

hysterical mutism The patient makes no effort to speak, but laryngeal function is normal and under **hypnosis** or powerful **suggestion** normal utterances can be achieved.

myoclonus A sudden spasm of the muscles, lifting and jerking the limbs. Can occur between **fits** in **epilepsy,** or with illnesses resulting from degeneration of brain cells. See also **nocturnal jerks.**

mystical experience   A feeling state experienced as unworldly; one which surpasses normal human description, explanation or understanding, and is felt to carry profound spiritual or other significance. In **psychiatry,** mystical experiences occur in **hysterical** illness and in the early stages of **schizophrenia.**

myxoedema   **Hypothyroidism** of the middle to later life usually of insidious onset with marked puffiness of the skin due to mucinous deposits. Physical features are those of hypothyroidism but with more commonly associated psychological accompaniments. Dullness of **personality, apathy,** fatigue, **memory** loss, including failure to register, can be associated with profound depression or a typical schizophrenic picture, in which **paranoid** elements tend to predominate; also frank **dementia** can supervene as can acute **confusion** and convulsive disorders, and **coma.**

nail biting   A **sign** of **nervousness** or tension. The most frequent habitual manipulation of the body occurring commonly throughout childhood and in some cases persisting into the beginning of adult life. Rarely of great psychopathological significance.

narcissism   A **psychoanalytic** term derived from the myth of Narcisus who fell in love with his own reflected image and was metamorphosed into the flower. **Freud** advanced his concept of narcissism as a development of his **libido** theory: the libido is withdrawn from its investment (**cathexis**) in other persons and becomes cathected onto the self. He postulated a state of primary narcissism at birth; the infant invests his libidinal energy only in the satisfaction of his own needs and self-preservation. As the infant develops, libido becomes attached to others, but a necessary amount of libido remains narcissistic throughout life. As a consequence of physical or psychic trauma in later life, libido may be withdrawn from other persons and reinvested in the body or self, and this state is termed secondary narcissism.

narcolepsy   A **syndrome** of sudden, almost irresistible brief attacks of **sleep** often associated with other sleep disorders such as sleep paralysis and **hallucinosis,** and with **cataplexy** and geloplegia (forced laughing attacks with falling). The cause is usually unknown but the condition can, rarely, be postencephalitic or due to other disorders of the brain stem.

narcosis   Unconsciousness induced by **sedative** or anaesthetic **drugs.**

narcotic drug   A substance which can induce drowsiness, **sleep,** stupefaction or insensibility according to its strength and the amount taken.

natural history The way a disease or disability evolves over time, uninfluenced by therapeutic intervention.

necrophilia A **sexual deviation** in which gratification is obtained from sexual contact with a dead person.

negative feeling Hostile and/or suspicious response to a person or situation.

negativism A tendency to manifest the opposite response to what is requested. May occur in **schizophrenia** as a direct **resistance** to what is seen as imposed demand. The individual does the opposite of what he is asked to do.

neo-Freudian Term referring to psychoanalysts who departed from **Freud's** position and gave more emphasis to cultural and interpersonal **behaviour,** in addition to intrapsychic experience, such as Karen **Horney**, Erich Fromm, Harry Stack **Sullivan** and Frieda Fromm-Reichman. The term is also imprecisely used to refer to the theories of these analysts and their followers, which differ considerably the one from the other.

neologism A new word which is meaningful to the patient who creates it, but is not readily understandable to others. It is classically described in **schizophrenia,** but can also occur in **dreams.**

nervous breakdown Common euphemism or exaggeration, with no precise meaning, used to signify any unwanted mental manifestation or reaction, lasting or transient, in dramatic or genteel manner of speaking.

nervous debility A colloquial expression usually meaning a state of tiredness or exhaustion, with lethargy rather than the over-excitability of **nervousness,** attributed to psychological causes.

nervousness A colloquial term indicating a state of general excitability or arousal, usually associated with apprehension or anticipatory **anxiety.** As a trait it indicates a proneness to **neurotic** responses or a chronic state of anxiety.

neurasthenia A **neurosis** characterized by abnormal fatigue, irritability, headache, depressed **mood, insomnia,** difficulty in concentrating and lack of capacity for enjoyment (**anhedonia**). It may follow or accompany an infection or exhaustion, or arise from continued emotional **stress.** The term was introduced in the United

States by psychologist G.M. Beard in 1869. In the 19th century it was used as a generic term but was regarded by **Freud** as an actual neurosis. During the early part of the 20th century various adjectival types were recognized, e.g. aviator's, postinfectious, professional, traumatic, tropical or war. Now in limited use to encompass cases in which the major feature is persistent fatigue.

neuroleptics A group of psychopharmacological agents which calm the patient without producing **sleep.** Included are several chemical classes of **drugs** such as the **phenothiazines,** the **butyrophenones** and the thioxanthines. All have a selective action to modify or alleviate **psychotic symptoms** such as restlessness and other psychomotor activity. Side-effects include lowering of blood pressure and the **extrapyramidal syndrome.** Used for **schizophrenia, manic** disorder and **organic confusional states.**

neurologist A medical practitioner specializing in **neurology.**

neurology That branch of medicine which deals with the study, diagnosis and treatment of disorders of the nervous system, including the brain, spinal cord and peripheral nerves.

neurosis (syn. psychoneurosis) **Mental illness** without any physical cause in which considerable **insight** is retained and reality **judgement** is intact (unlike the **psychoses**). The patient's **behaviour** and thinking are maladaptive and cause suffering, but usually remain in socially acceptable limits. Only part of the **personality** is disorganized. Diagnosed when one of the charactersitic **syndromes** of neurosis is present (**anxiety, obsessional, depressive, hysterical** and **phobic** types). Most often precipitated by an environmental setback of special symbolic significance to the patient, who may have been predisposed to illness by an early corresponding psychological setback during childhood.

accident neurosis A variant of **hysterical neurosis** most commonly, following an accident or injury, when compensation is being sought. More common after injury to the head than to other sites. May be accompanied, but rarely, by **postconcussional syndrome.** *See also* **neurosis, compensation.**

anxiety neurosis An illness characterized by a morbid state of **fear** and apprehension, associated with other unpleasant **mood** and physical **symptoms** like palpitations, difficulty in breathing, dizziness etc. The **anxiety** usually occurs without there being any external frightening stimulus, and may amount to extreme panic. According to **DSM-III,** subdivided into generalized anxiety disorder (anxiety symptoms without **panic attacks**) and panic disorder (recurrent panic attacks).

cardiac neurosis A morbid preoccupation with **symptoms,** thought by the sufferer to refer to the heart, and a **fear** of heart disease without any physical abnormalities. A particular variant, disordered action of the heart (DAH), effort **syndrome** or Da Costa's syndrome, is characterized by palpitations, shortness of breath and subjective discomfort following slight exertion and was first recognized in the American Civil War but came to prominence during the First World War. According to **DSM-III,** would be considered **hypochondriasis.**

compensation neurosis **Neurotic** disability following an accident or illness which is reinforced by the prospect of financial compensation. *See also* **neurosis.**

depressive neurosis A reactive **depressive illness** is to be differentiated from endogenous **depressive illness.** It is usually regarded as a response to **stress,** and the **symptoms** may disappear if the patient is in a protected environment or the stress removed. The absence of physical symptoms e.g. poor appetite, fatigue, with the, presence of other **neurotic** features and responsiveness of **mood** distinguish neurotic depressive illness from the major depressive disorders.

hysterical conversion neurosis A **syndrome** in which there is a loss of or alteration in bodily functioning that suggests physical disorder, but which instead is apparently an expression of a psychological **conflict** or need of which the patient is unaware. Common **symptoms** are paralysis, blindness and co-ordination disturbances such as **tremors,** numbness, vomiting etc. The illness can be monosymptomatic such as loss of voice **(aphonia),** or differing symptoms can occur in succession; recurrent attacks of the disorder can occur. To be differentiated from **hysterical personality disorder.**

hysterical dissociative neurosis A group of **neurotic** disorders in which the patient suffers a temporary alteration in the level of awareness, and by means of **dissociation** splits off a part of **consciousness,** and hence suffers from **memory** loss **(amnesia), fugues** or multiple **personality.**

obsessional neurosis (syn. compulsive neurosis, obsessive-compulsive neurosis) A neurosis in which the predominant **symptoms** are **obsessions,** repetitive **thoughts,** ideas or images, and compulsive **behaviour.** The outstanding symptom is a feeling of subjective **compulsion,** which the sufferer feels must be resisted, to carry out some action, to dwell upon an idea, to recall an experience or to ruminate on an abstract topic. The urge or idea is recognized as irrational and alien to the **personality,** yet as coming from within the self. Obsessional or compulsive actions may be quasi-**ritual** performances which are designed to relieve **anxiety** but which, if resisted, generate intense anxiety.

occupational neurosis   A psychologically determined disability affecting those actions which are essential to the performance of the patient's occupation, such as **writer's cramp.** *See also* **occupational cramp.**

phobic neurosis   *See* **phobic illness.**

traumatic neurosis   A **syndrome** developed following exposure to a psychologically stressful situation, or events that are generally outside the normal range of human experience such as **rape,** assault, torture, military combat. The characteristic **symptoms** include re-experiencing the traumatic events in recurrent **dreams** or intrusive memories, a numbing of general responsiveness to the external world, exaggerated startle reaction or other signs of **anxiety,** and **sleep** disturbance. In **DSM-III,** called post-traumatic stress disorder.

war neurosis   (syn. battle neurosis, combat neurosis, **shell shock**) An acute **traumatic neurosis** occurring as a consequence of exposure to the risks of battle. Often occurs following chronic exposure to situations of high risk, particularly where physical casualties occur among immediate companions. Post-traumatic stress disorder is the relevent **DSM-III** term.

neurosyphilis   (syn. **general paresis**) Refers to the tertiary stage of the syphilitic process in the brain resulting in psychological change, **dementia** or localized neurological disorder. Famous patients include Maupassant and Delius, and Ibsen gave the affliction to Oswald Alving in "Ghosts".

neurotic   Relating to a **neurosis** or a person suffering from a neurosis. 1. A departure from normal which is unhealthy but is not **organic** or **psychotic,** and can be explained in psychological terms. 2. A colloquial expression, often pejorative, implying highly strung, tense, nervy or over-responsive **behaviour** which is usually explicable in psychological terms. In **DSM-III,** a descriptive term for a mental disorder in which the predominant disturbance is a **symptom** or group of symptoms distressing to the individual and recognized by him or her as unacceptable and alien. **Reality testing** is intact and there is no demonstrable organic cause or factor.

neurotic depressive state   *See* **neurosis, depressive.**

neurotransmitter   A chemical substance contained in nerve endings to transmit impulses across the minute gaps between the nerves, and from them to the muscles or glands they supply.

Nietzsche, Friedrich (1844–1900)   German philosopher, born in Leipzig, the son of a Lutheran clergyman. Appointed to the Chair of Classical Philology at Basle at age 24 where he remained until 1871 when illness forced his resignation. He was disabled by severe psychiatric illness during the last 11 years of his life. In early works Nietzsche developed a nihilistic philosophy in which he asserted the death of God, of rationality, and of accepted moral values. In response to the absence of certainty, Nietzsche proposed a self-directed, life-affirming existence to be seen as an opportunity to become 'aeronauts of the spirit'; to 'live dangerously'; and to 'build cities on the sides of volcanoes'. The ideal aspiration of man should be towards becoming a 'superman', and 'warrior of ideas'. The 'will to power' has often been misunderstood as a call to militarism and inhumane authoritarianism, not Nietzsche's intention; probably best understood as an early and influential version of 'becoming' (**Dasein**) in **existential** terms: men may make their lives by their willed actions, rather than by submitting passively to unvalidated external mores and demands.

night terrors   *(pavor nocturnus)* A form of **sleep** disturbance consisting of frightening **dreams** in children while asleep, leading to extreme terror and **confusion**. Different from **nightmares** in that no part of the dream is recalled on awakening.

nightmare   A common and frightening **dream** experience of occasional occurrence in young children. The child wakes in **fear** and can usually remember vividly some of the dream content.

nihilism   Strictly a doctrine that denies moral principles and social obligations, or an extreme anarchistic approach. In **psychiatry** it tends to be applied to a state in which the individual has a subjective experience of dissolution of himself or of the outside world. *See also* **Cotard's syndrome; delusion, nihilistic.**

noctambulism   *See* **somnambulism.**

nocturnal jerks   Many normal people experience jerks, often of the whole body, during the phase of going to **sleep** (more rarely on waking). The underlying neurophysiological mechanism is uncertain. More rarely, some **epileptics** have myoclonic jerks during sleep which may waken the sufferer. *See also* **myoclonus.**

nominal aphasia   *See* **aphasia.**

non-accidental injury   Young children, especially babies are occasionally injured by those looking after them, usually their parents. The injuries are usually physical (for example beatings, burnings) but the term is extended to include the giving of poison, dangerous drugs, sexual abuse, starvation and any other physical assault. A proportion of the children so damaged appear to be in some way already abnormal, physically and/or mentally, thereby posing a problem of being more difficult to be looked after than normal children. The persons responsible for inflicting the injuries are also often themselves psychologically disturbed. Recognition for what they are is often difficult as is also the subsequent management of the social situation.

noradrenaline *See* **brain amines.**

normality 1. A statistical average, e.g. normal **intelligence.** 2. An absence of pathology, e.g. normal health. 3. That which society deems acceptable; a pragmatic norm.

  actuarial normality The statistical average.

  ideal normality *See* **normality,** 2.

nosology The science of the classification of diseases.

nutritional disorders An imprecise term denoting either the conditions caused by dietary deficiency, or those disorders of eating caused by psychological pressures, i.e. **obesity, anorexia nervosa, bulimia.**

nymphomania (obs.) Abnormally heightened sexual desire in a woman.

obesity The condition of being excessively stout or corpulent, considered present when the person weighs 20 per cent more than the accepted weight for his height and build. The excess fat, mostly in the tissues under the skin, results from more food intake than is required for the energy expended by daily activity. There can be hormonal disorder as a contributing cause.

obfuscation The presentation of information in such a way so as to confuse or mislead.

object relation The relation of a person to the inner representation in his mind of another. In **psychoanalysis,** object relations theory refers to the psychological internalization of others, these inner structures forming mental part-objects (e.g. good mother) in constituting the **psyche.**

obsession An intrusive, unwelcome **thought** or feeling, often absurd and incongruous, resisted by the individual but recognized by him

occupational cramp

as coming from within himself. May take the form of repetitive self-searching or questioning (**rumination**) or imperative urges to count monotonously. *See also* **compulsion.**

occupational cramp   A psychologically caused spasm of muscles preventing the patient from carrying out his occupation, such as **writer's cramp**, clerical worker's hands, musician's cramp etc. Often due to **conflict,** such as that between dutiful performance of work on the one hand and distaste or fear on the other.

occupational neurosis   *See* **occupational cramp.**

occupational therapy   Profession directed to **rehabilitation,** treatment and diversion through handicrafts (carpentry, pottery, painting, etc.), expressive activities such as **psychodrama,** music and poetry-reading, industrial therapy and housecraft, under the direction of an occupational therapist in hospitals or day centres.

oceanic feeling   In **psychoanalysis,** a mystical, expansive **emotion.** According to **Freud, regression** to an early **ego** state reviving the experience of the infant at the breast before ego has been differentiated from external reality.

oculogyric crisis   A **symptom** of idiopathic or drug-induced **Parkinsonism,** where the eyeball is rotated upwards by spasm of the ocular muscles.

oedipal stage   The period of **personality development** between three and five years of age when the child comes to grasp the anatomical difference between the sexes, and is intensely curious about the facts of procreation and the implications of gender. According to **psychoanalysis,** the child at this stage establishes inner psychological representations of his parents, which determine his sexual role and preferences in adulthood. *See also* **complex, Oedipus, personality development, psychic ontogeny.**

Oedipus complex   *See* **complex.**

oligophrenia   *See* **mental retardation.**

onanism   (obs.) Term meaning either **masturbation** or sexual intercourse interrupted before ejaculation, depending on one's biblical interpretation of the 'sins of Onan', who 'spilt his seed upon the ground'.

oneirism   Dreamlike state occurring when the person is awake.

oneiroid   Dreamlike, the term usually being applied not to **organic** disturbances of **consciousness,** as in **confusional states,** but to **withdrawal** so that the patient objectively seems out of touch. Profound **psychotic** episodes have sometimes been called **oneirophrenia;** on recovery patients usually have a patchy **amnesia** but may recall vivid and fantastic **hallucinations.**

oneirophrenia   A **dreamlike** state, with a good outcome, sometimes caused by physical illness. Most often a **functional** psychiatric illness, of atypical schizophrenic type. **Thought disorder** and alterations and incongruities of **mood** occur, but there is **clouding** of **consciousness** (not a characteristic feature of **schizophrenia).**

ontology   The study and theory of the nature of being or existence.

ontogeny   Origin and development of an individual, in contrast to phylogeny, the development of the species.

psychic ontogeny   In **psychoanalysis,** phases of **personality development** through the psychosocial stages differentiated into **oral, anal, genital** and **latency stages** during childhood.

opiates   **Narcotic** and **analgesic drugs** obtained from the dried juice of the unripe seed capsule of the poppy, *Papaver somniferum.* **Morphine** is the principal naturally-ocurring alkaloid; others include codeine, thebaine, papaverine and noscapine. Diacetylmorphine **(heroin)** is easily made from morphine, and hydromorphine, oxymorphone, hydrocodone and oxycodone can also be made by modifying the morphine molecule.

opioid   Any natural or synthetic **drug** that has **morphine**-like pharmacological actions. The term is used interchangeably with **narcotic analgesic,** and drugs of this group are all effective in the relief of pain but carry the risk of physical and psychological **dependence.**

opisthotonus   A condition of gross arching of the back due to generalized spasm of the body musculature. It occurs with strychnine poisoning, tetanus, in association with profound jaundice in the newborn, and cerebellar **fits.** Very similar states can be seen in severe **hysterical neurosis,** sometimes called arc de cercle.

oral stage   In **psychoanalysis** the first **pregenital** stage of infantile psychosocial development. It is usually divided into an oral- dependent period, characterized by sucking and other activities associated with feeding, and an oral-aggressive or oral-sadistic period, during

organic

which the infant becomes more active and assertive. The stage is associated in later life with the oral personality, including excessive **dependence** and demands for **attention** and support from other people.

organic   Of a disorder associated with changes in an organ, e.g. the brain. The changes can be transient as in **delirium** due to **drugs** or infection (e.g. **meningitis)**, or permanent as in **senile dementia.** cf. **functional.**

orgasm   A neurophysiological event which may occur during sexual arousal, characterized by a peak of pleasurable sensation and generalized muscle tension, both clonic and tonic, and followed by a marked release of tension and reduction of arousal. In postpubertal males it is normally accompanied by seminal emission, which results in ejaculation.

orientation   Awareness of oneself in time, space, place and person. Impaired in physical brain disturbance (**delirium** and **dementia),** and in toxic states such as occur with infection and by **drugs,** etc.

orthopsychiatry   Vague concept related to mental hygiene and the prevention of mental and emotional disorder by attention to healthy development.

Othello syndrome   *See* **jealousy, delusional.**

overcompensation   One of the **defence mechanisms,** and a psychological maladjustment whereby the person tries to overcome or conceal a real or imagined failing or inferiority by undue manifestation of the opposite attribute, e.g. a timid person may behave threateningly, or a man fearing he is effeminate can behave in an overassertively masculine way.

overdetermination   In **psychoanalysis,** many factors operating together to bring about preferences in personal relationships, patterns of **behaviour, neurosis** and other developments of the **personality.**

overeating   Eating too much or eating to excess; a common pattern of **behaviour** in affluent society where the caloric intake often grossly exceeds that required for normal daily activity. **Eating disorders** of various kinds may be associated with regular or intermittent overeating. *See also* **anorexia nervosa; bulimia.**

112

overvalued idea Strongly held false **belief** developing comprehensibly out of a given **personality** and life situation. May occur in both healthy and mentally disordered individuals (e.g. in the latter, when the individual believes wrongly that he stinks).

paederast Someone who practices **sodomy**; usually confined to anal intercourse with boys.

paedophilia Sexual attraction to children, usually as the preferred age of sexual partner. A paedophiliac may be attracted particularly to boys, to girls or to either sex. Such preferences in women are very unusual.

pain, atypical A variable dull, throbbing, aching or boring pain which does not respond to **analgesics** or correspond to anatomical distributions and may be a depressive equivalent. This is well recognized among the atypical facial neuralgias where such pain may respond to **antidepressant** treatment.

palilalia The involuntary repitition of words or phrases e.g. 'Where is my pen, is my pen, is my pen?': especially a feature of postencephalitic **Parkinsonism.**

panic attacks An acute sense of overwhelming dread usually of abrupt onset and usually self-limiting, lasting from seconds to hours. There is an explosive **autonomic** arousal state with palpitations, pallor, dizziness, sweating, tremulousness, nausea and a desire to evacuate bowels and bladder. The accompanying affect of **fear** results in restlessness and a desire to escape. **Depersonalization** and **derealization** may supervene. After the attack the patient feels exhausted.

panic disorder *See* **neurosis, anxiety.**

paradoxical interpretation *See* **interpretation.**

paradoxical sleep *See* **sleep.**

paraesthesia Subjective cutaneous sensation usually of numbness and tingling, sometimes associated with actual partial sensory loss to touch and pain. There are a variety of causes; the condition is often transient and localized as a result of pressure on peripheral nerves.

paralysis agitans Term for the condition better known as **Parkinsonism.**

paramnesia   A disorder of **memory** in which there is a distortion or falsification of **recall.** Includes retrospective falsification, retrospective **delusions** and delusional memories, and **confabulation.**

paranoia   A rare and chronic mental disorder characterized by the emergence of **paranoid delusions** organized into a more or less coherent system, without other marked **symptoms** of psychiatric illness such as **hallucinations** or **mood** disturbance.

paranoid delusions   *See* delusions, paranoid.

paranoid illness   An acute **paranoid psychosis** seemingly precipitated by emotional **stress.**

paranoid symptom   Features of a mental state characterized by the presence of **delusions.** May include morbid suspicion, persecution **beliefs,** or ideas of grandeur.

paraphrenia   A **psychotic** condition, often a subtype of **schizophrenia,** characterized by absurd **delusions** but well-preserved social function and little, if any, deterioration even after years of illness. Occurs in middle age, while late paraphrenia is applied to predominantly **paranoid** delusions of a highly systemized kind (e.g. that the neighbours are plotting against the patient) occurring in old age.

parapraxis   Slips of the tongue which, according to **psychoanalytic theory,** signify the true feelings, wishes or **thoughts** of the speaker buried in the non-reporting part of the **mind** or the **unconscious** because of the action of the **superego** or censor. e.g. The professor who, when concerned and threatened by his colleagues at a symposium, says on opening the meeting 'I now declare this meeting closed'.

parapsychology   That branch of **psychology** concerned with **extrasensory perception** (ESP), **telepathy** and other mental processes usually regarded as outside the normal abilities of man (and animals).

parasuicide   *See* suicide attempt.

parasympathetic nervous system   The division of the **autonomic nervous system,** confined to the head, neck and trunk, held to be primarily concerned with restorative function, using acetylcholine as a **neurotransmitter** at the target organs.

pareidolia   **Illusions** which may occur in normal people where there is full **insight** and which may be enhanced by increased **attention,** e.g. seeing pictures in the fire or in clouds etc.

Parkinsonism   Disorder characterized by a coarse **tremor** of the head and limbs, **rigidity** and expressionless face, due to disease or impairment, e.g. by drugs such as **phenothiazines,** of the basal ganglia of the brain. Also referred to as the **extrapyramidal reaction**. When drug-induced, usually stops if the medication is withdrawn or the dose lessened.

passivity feelings   Experience of direct invasive influence from outside on **thought,** feelings or actions. A cardinal **symptom** of **schizophrenia** in **Schneider's** symptoms of the first rank.

Patau's syndrome   A congenital condition characterised by microcephaly, **mental retardation** and a variety of structural abnormalities, including abnormal facies, cleft lip and palate and undecended testes. It results from an autosomal chromosome abnormality, trisomy 15. *See also* **chromosome anomalies.**

pathogenic event   An event believed to play a substantial role in the causation of a pathological state. e.g. After being told by his wife that she is leaving him, the husband may become ill with a **depressive neurosis.**

pathognomonic   A **symptom** or **sign** that is characteristic of a particular disease state, in the sense that its presence allows firm diagnosis of the illness.

pathological lying   A tendency to utter false statements or declarations which often serve no clear purpose. May be a manifestation of **personality disorder.** *See also* **pseudologia fantastica.**

Pavlov, Ivan Petrovitch (1849–1936)   Russian physiologist and Nobel prize winner in 1904. His primary contribution was to the theory and study of reflexes: the class of innate reflexes, such as salivation caused by the presentation of food, he termed unconditioned reflexes. **Conditioned reflexes** are formed when an independent sensory stimulus (such as a bell ringing), not usually able to elicit the response repeatedly accompanies the presentation of food and salivation. The ringing is then termed a conditioned stimulus, and the salivation which occurs in response to it is termed a **conditioned reflex**. Pavlov held that this mechanism, rather than **instinct**, is the basis of all **behaviour**. Those reflexes that are rewarded (reinforced) persist. Those that are punished or not rein-

Penfield, Wilder G. (1891–1976)

forced are extinguished. The sensory cues of conditioned reflexes constitute a primary signalling system. In man verbal cues (language) form a secondary signalling system, capable of eliciting a vast range of complex behaviour. Pavlov's clinical theories are derived directly from his neural reflexology: **neuroses** and **psychoses** are an expression of a functional incapacity of the malfunctioning brain hemispheres. His theories have had a strong influence on psychiatric theory and practice in the Soviet Union and he is a major source of theory for **behaviour therapy**.

Penfield, Wilder G. (1891–1976) Canadian neurosurgeon and author at McGill University, his interests in cerebral localization and surgical treatment of **epilepsy** led to the discovery that stimulation of discrete areas of the cortex in conscious subjects could elicit emotional responses and **recall** of past experiences.

penis envy In **psychoanalytic theory,** a common component of the **genital stage** of psychosocial development, when the penis becomes a focus of interest to children of both sexes. Often extended to include **personality** traits in women, related to envy of the male role.

percept The mental product of the act of perceiving; a meaningful sensation possessing full objective reality for the individual. It may constitute a response to an outside stimulus (true percept) or it may arise in the absence of such stimulation (false percept, e.g. **hallucination**).

perception The act of experiencing a **percept.**

perceptual deprivation (syn. sensory deprivation) A state of sensory **isolation** or information deficit. Can be induced experimentally by isolating the individual in a darkened vibration-free room or immersed in a water tank. The effects resemble **brainwashing** and produce an intense desire for stimulation, increased **suggestibility,** impaired **thinking, depressed mood,** a sense of oppression and, in extreme cases, **confusion, hallucinations** and **delusions.**

perplexity A morbid state in which there is subjective bewilderment with a sense of puzzling change in the environment. Objectively the patient may be distractible with a hint of **clouding** of **consciousness.** Found in **organic** states, **schizophrenia** of acute onset and puerperal **psychoses.**

perseveration The continuation of a motor or verbal response, originally appropriate to a stimulus, past the point where utility ends.

persona   The face one presents to the world. In Greek drama, a mask. Term of **Jung** for the overt attitudes and **behaviour** of an individual in everyday life.

personal history   As part of the psychiatric assessment, a recorded description of the principal events of an individual's life. Includes data pertaining to birth, early development and experiences, education, illnesses, occupations, sexual inclinations and practice, marital experiences, family life, living circumstances, and other aspects of personal functioning.

personal identity   Self-awareness; recognition of personal uniqueness and integrity as a continuous being throughout the stages of the life cycle; the features which constitute the uniqueness of the individual.

personality   An inexact term for the sum total of a person's actions and reactions, characteristic of his **behaviour,** differentiating one individual from another. Can be approached in terms of categories (e.g. **normal, hysterical, schizoid** etc.) or of dimensions (e.g. **extraversion,** neuroticism etc.).

anal personality   Personality with prominent traits of orderliness, parsimony and obstinacy. In **psychoanalytic theory,** this personality arises from fixation at the **anal stage** of development in infancy.

cycloid personality   Personality showing tendency to swings of **mood** and energy, either high or low.

cyclothymic personality   *See* **personality, cycloid.**

dependent personality   Personality showing tendency to lean on others for protection, advice, guidance and support. Self-esteem is usually low and the individual may subordinate his or her own needs to those of others on whom he or she is dependent.

dual or multiple personality   An hysterical dissociative **neurosis** where contrasting personalities may present in the same individual, each 'person' being seemingly unaware of the existence of the other(s). The original or primary personality coexists or alternates with another relatively distinct and separate secondary (or tertiary etc.) personality which appears to lead a distinct existence. Examples in fiction are Dr. Jekyll and Mr. Hyde, and in the clinical literature Morton Prince's case of Miss Beauchamp, and Cleckley and Thigpen's case of Eve.

eccentric personality   Personality showing non-specific socially unusual **behaviour.**

epileptic personality (obs.) Chronic personality disorders (slowness, stickiness of **thinking, paranoid** tendencies, moodiness, irritability, etc.) said to be typical of persons with **epilepsy** but in fact found in a minority of such persons (usually with chronic temporal seizures) and multifactorial in origin.

histrionic personality Personality showing excessive but shifting and labile emotional responses with a tendency to seek attention. In **DSM III**, syn. for **hysterical personality disorder.**

immature personality Imprecise term for personality exhibiting traits of **dependence,** inclined to be excessively demanding and manifesting emotional responses of a childish nature.

inadequate personality Personality lacking physical and emotional stamina and manifesting poor adaptation in many sectors of life.

multiple personality *See* **personality, dual.**

normal personality 1. A person in whom no evidence of abnormality is present. 2. Empirical definition used for research purposes in **epidemiology,** e.g. somebody who has not seen a **psychiatrist** nor consulted a doctor with a nervous ailment during the preceding year. 3. An ideal concept conveying the aspiration towards a desired state, e.g. 'a state of complete physical, mental and social well-being' (World Health Organization). 4. A statistical definition implying that state characterizing most people contained in the community of which the person is a member. 5. Of a person who has adequately negotiated all the formative stages constituting **personality development** and arrived at a state of maturity. 6. One free of clinically evident **personality disorder.**

obsessional personality A personality type inclined to caution, tidiness, meticulousness and over-conscientiousness often with a degree of **rigidity.**

oral personality *See* oral stage.

personality development Evolution of the personality from infancy onwards through stages which can each be identified, given the basic constitution and the psychosocial environment in which the individual develops. Numerous theories have been advanced about such evolution, e.g. by **Freud, Sullivan, Erikson** etc.

personality disorder Disturbance of personality manifesting as fixed maladaptive patterns of **behaviour** continuing throughout most of adult life. The deviation leads the person to suffer, or causes others to suffer. It can be identified on the basis of trait disturbances, e.g. excessive hostility, undue **dependence** and passivity, or excessive scrupulousness, or on the basis of repetitive disturbance in personal relationships.

anankastic personality disorder   *See* **personality disorder, obsessional.**

antisocial personality disorder   *See* **personality disorder, sociopathic.**

dependent personality disorder   Refers to indivduals who are not self- reliant but passively depend on others to make decisions for them, support them emotionally and meet their material needs. They comply passively with the wishes of others and respond inadequately to the demands of daily life. The essential feature is getting others to assume responsibility for the major areas of one's life.

explosive personality disorder   Personality disorder characterized by instability of **mood** with sudden outbursts of **emotion** and extreme rage reactions. Sometimes seen in those with **epilepsy.** The **ICD-9** definition stresses that aggressive outbursts, verbal or physical, cannot readily be controlled by the person, who is not otherwise prone to **antisocial behaviour.**

hysterical personality disorder   A disorder of persons who are habitually inclined to dramatize themselves and situations and whose **affects** are labile and shallow. Dependency and a morbid craving for **attention** are additional features. *See also* **personality, histrionic**

narcissistic personality disorder   Personality disorder of abnormal people with unwarranted self-importance or sense of uniqueness, greatly distressed when their self-esteem is threatened, and whose relationships with others are characterized by exploitiveness, entitlement and vacillation between extremes of over-idealization and devaluation. In addition, there may be features of **borderline state, hysterical personality disorder** or **sociopathy.** A category of diagnosis used in the United States (**DSM- III**).

obsessional personality disorder   A disorder of persons manifesting strong insecure feelings and liable to **ambivalence.** Commonly associated features include morbid sensitivity, excessive orderliness, overconscientionsness, punctuality, and need for sameness.

paranoid personality disorder   Personality with a pervasive and unwarranted suspiciousness and mistrust of people. There is hypersensitivity to criticism and often pathological **jealousy.**

passive personality disorder   Refers to individuals who are not competent nor effective, but have a weak inadequate response to life demands, and who are readily liable to **dependence** on others with an excessive compliance with their wishes.

passive-aggressive personality disorder A personality disorder in which there is **resistance,** expressed indirectly, to demands for adequate performance in both occupational and social functioning. The resistance is expressed through such **symptoms** as procrastination, stubbornness and quasi-intentional inefficiency.

psychopathic personality disorder *See* **personality disorder, sociopathic.**

schizoid personality disorder Personality with a defect in the capacity to form social relations, evidenced by the absence of warm, tender feelings for others and indifference to praise, criticism, and the feelings of others. In **DSM-III** distinguished from **schizotypal personality disorder.**

schizotypal personality disorder A diagnostic category used in the United States (**DSM-III**) for patients who have oddities of **thought, perception,** speech and **behaviour** that are not severe enough to meet the criteria for **schizophrenia.** In other diagnostic systems these disorders might be classified as **borderline, latent** or **pseudoneurotic** schizophrenia.

sociopathic personality disorder, sociopathy. Personality disorder of severe degree, present from an early age, the person harming himself and others through gross impairment in personal relationships. Characterized by failure to learn from mistakes, emotional unconcern sometimes amounting to callousness, demand for immediate gratification of needs and impulses, extreme exploitation of others, absence of **guilt** for **antisocial** acts and disregard for social obligations. Aggressiveness and irresponsibility lead to trouble with the law. Some are not hostile and assaultative but grossly passive and dependent. Response to efforts at treatment is poor, although troublesomeness often improves with ageing. Antisocial personality disorder in **DSM-III.**

persuasion 1. The induction of a **belief** or attitude by the clinician, sometimes employed as a component of **psychotherapy.** 2. The practice of inducing change in an individual's mental state by directly urging the value or benefits of a particular **behaviour** or point of view.

perversion A term used in the past to describe any form of abnormal sexual **behaviour.** It is now seldom used by **psychiatrists** because of its clearly judgmental and pejorative meaning. It remains a technical term within **psychoanalysis.** *See also* **sexual deviation.**

PET scan   *See* **positron emission tomography.**

petrol sniffing   A form of **solvent abuse** occurring most commonly when alcohol or other intoxicants are not available, but some episodic use by young people is reported. Inhalation is often directly from the filler tubes of vehicle petrol tanks. This form of solvent abuse carries the additional long-term hazard of lead poisoning.

phaeochromocytoma   A tumour of the adrenal medulla, an endocrine gland above the kidney, which produces surges of noradrenaline or adrenaline, causing tachycardia, feelings of **anxiety** and changes in blood pressure.

phallic stage   In **psychoanalytic theory,** the stage reached in the fourth and fifth year, after the **anal** and before the **Oedipal stage,** when the child is preoccupied with his penis, its functions and its potency, and associated with **masturbation** fantasies. In boys **castration anxiety** and in girls **penis envy** are regarded as closely related. A phallic character is viewed as a person with **fixation** on sexual **behaviour** as a display of potency, in contrast to a genital character who views it as sharing in a relationship.

phantasy   *See* **fantasy.**

phantom limb   Following amputation of a limb, neuronal activity in the stump is experienced as occurring in the lost limb itself. Pain is a particular and intractable problem responding very poorly to **analgesics.**

phenomenology   In **psychiatry,** the clinical method giving precedence to the patient's actual experiences, the clinician avoiding preconceived theories but attending meticulously to the patient's communications about his own subjective state. Derives from **Husserl's** philosophy of attending to things themselves, first applied to psychiatry by Karl **Jaspers** in his book *General Psychopathology* (1913).

phenothiazines   The generic term for a series of **neuroleptic** compounds, based on the same parent molecule, used widely in **psychiatry** as antipsychotic **drugs.**

phenotype   The observable attributes of an individual, brought about by the interaction of the **genes** he has inherited (**genotype**) and his environment and life circumstances.

phenylketonuria   **Mental retardation** inherited as an autosomal recessive trait, with fair skin and hair, and a history of **convulsions** due to a deficiency of phenylalanine 4-monooxygenase so that phenylpyruvic acid appears in the blood and urine. The condition is now rarely untreated as it is usually detected by screening at birth. Increasing experience and knowledge have led to the discovery of aberrant forms.

phobia   Excessive **fear** and morbid dread when in contact with particular objects or situations which are not ordinarily a source of danger, e.g. dogs, air travel, enclosed spaces. Sufferers avoid the objects of their dread, or situations which make them anxious.

phobic illness   Form of **neurosis** in which **phobia** is the chief **symptom.** Types include **agoraphobia, claustrophobia,** social phobia (fear of being with people) and specific phobias (e.g. of cats, thunder, heights, sharp knives etc.). Treatment is by **behaviour therapy (desensitization, flooding), psychotherapy** or drugs such as **benzodiazepines.**

photopsia   The sensation of flashes or sparks of light which can occur in a wide variety of disorders of the visual system, located from the retina of the eye to the visual cortex of the brain.

phrenology   An outmoded study in which it was presumed that the aspects of **personality** resided in specific areas of the brain. The degree to which these parts of the brain were developed was thought to be reflected in the contours of the skull, which was studied and described in attempts to understand the person.

physical abstinence syndrome   Those **symptoms** which result from the **withdrawal** of a **drug** or drugs and which vary according to the individual drug. In mildest form there may be only paroxysmal abnormalities in the **EEG** but tremulousness, **anxiety,** weakness, restlessness and **insomnia** are common. Grand mal seizures and **delirium** occur in severe cases of **central nervous system** depressant withdrawal. *See also* **withdrawal symptoms.**

physical dependence capacity   The ability of a **drug** to act as a substitute for another upon which an organism has been made physically dependent, i.e. to suppress abstinence phenomena that would otherwise develop after abrupt withdrawal of the original dependence-producing drug; e.g. **methadone** in the treatment of **opiate addiction.**

physique   Body build in relation to **mental illness** was explored by **Kretschmer,** who advanced the view that when those with **pyknic** build became ill they tend to have **manic-depressive psychosis,** while the **asthenic** build (tall, thin, with little fat) is associated with

schizoid personality disorder and **schizophrenia.** Sheldon later differentiated the mesomorph (athletic), the endomorph (corresponding to the pyknic) and the ectomorph (corresponding to the asthenic). *See also* **typology.**

Piaget, Jean (1896–1979)   Swiss developmental psychologist, who described an **epigenetic** model of cognitive development proceeding from the concrete, particular, alogical, subjective mode of early infancy through intermediate stages to the capacity for general logical, abstract, symbolic thought in maturity. The first stage 'the sensorimotor period' is essentially reflexive. The next stage 'the preoperational stage' sees the beginning of symbolic **thought,** which is developed in the stage of 'concrete operations', during which numbers, and logical classes, are understood and manipulated. The stage of 'formal operations' characterizes **puberty** and **adolescence** and encompasses the capacity for true logical thought and the making of testable hypotheses. The primary units of **cognition** and response to the environment are 'schemata' which are organizations of behaviour relevant to each other. Schemata are derived from the constant processes of **'assimilation'** and **'accommodation'.** Assimilation is the process of taking in data from the environment. The new data have to be constantly incorporated into the pre-existing schemata, and in turn the schemata must change or 'accommodate' the newly assimilated data.

pica   Dirt eating, usually persistent; a **symptom** sometimes in mentally retarded children.

Pick's disease   This form of **presenile dementia** with an age of onset usually between 50 and 60 differs from **Alzheimer's disease** in that the early stages are characterized by disinhibition, tactless and insensitive social **behaviour,** and other features of **personality** change such as sexual misdemeanour, stealing and acts of cruelty. These changes, as also the **apathy,** fatuous **mood,** deterioration of personal habits, lack of **insight,** arise from the predominantly frontal localization of **brain damage** in the early stages. **Perseveration** of speech, **apraxia, agnosia,** and the disturbance of gait and muscle tone may appear at a later stage but are more pronounced in and characteristic of Alzheimer's disease. The condition proves rapidly fatal and at postmortem the brain shows shrinkage, but with damage selectively severe in the frontal and temporal lobes. Microscopic examination shows loss of brain cortical cells, and often distended oval-shaped 'balloon cells' which are characteristic.

Pinel, Philippe (1745–1826)   French physician and psychiatrist noted for his considerate and liberal approach to treatment of the

insane and for his scientifically oriented treatise on insanity. Historically celebrated for freeing the mentally ill from their chains at the
Bicêtre Hospital in 1787 where they had been kept by keepers with
whips and dogs. Regarded by some as the father of **psychiatry**, his
name is associated with moral i.e. humane treatment and the beginnings of **asylum** reform.

placebo   An inert tablet or capsule, sometimes prepared to appear
identical to a **drug** being tested in a clinical trial, and given under
double-blind conditions to minimize non-specific factors in attitudes
of the patient and the doctor to the treatment.

placebo effect (or **response**)   Physical and psychological benefits
and unfavourable reactions depending on the patient's expectations,
and the doctor's **behaviour,** and not on the treatment itself.

play therapy   The use of common childhood activities, toys, etc. by a
psychotherapist (usually of dynamic not behavioural orientation)
for treatment, especially of young children unable to communicate
verbally. The child **psychiatrist** or lay therapist provides a sand
tray, running water, containers, dolls and other toys, and watches as
the child plays, drawing inferences or making **interpretations** of the
play situations or events the child devises. The latter may be taken as
symbolic representations e.g. of **conflicts** or tensions in the parental
home, or of frustrations the child experiences in the family.

pleasure principle   **Psychoanalytic** term; the tendency towards
gratification of needs and the avoidance of pain and delay of
satisfaction; the characteristic mode of the **libido** of the immature
psyche. However, the pressure for immediate satisfaction is
modified by the demands of the external world. Thus, the pleasure
principle contains the demands of the **id** and is constrained by the
reality principle. '...the pleasure principle represents the claims of
the libido, and that modification of it, the reality principle, the
influence of the outer world' (**Freud**).

porphyria   A metabolic abnormality in which porphyrin metabolism
is disrupted, resulting in increased excretion of uroporphyrin and
related compounds in the urine, showing up as a purple colour when
the urine is exposed to light. Inborn errors of metabolism may be the
primary cause but **drugs** such as **barbiturates** may exacerbate or
trigger the **syndrome,** which consists of abdominal pain, photosen-
sitivity, **confusional states,** hypertrichosis and haemolytic
anaemia. One form is intermittent.

positive feeling   Warm spontaneous **affective** response.

positron emission tomography (PET scan)   One of the new imaging techniques to investigate the brain. *See also* **EMI scan, regional cerebral blood flow.**

possession   Derangement of the **mind,** ascribed to intrusion by an alien spirit. For centuries possession by the devil or by demons was considered the cause of insanity, and exorcism was practised as a cure. These states and their presumed cause remain very common in the East, Africa and the developing countries generally.

postconcussional symptoms   Following **concussion** patients may develop a wide variety of disorders. Some can be related to probable brain stem damage, e.g. tinnitus, hyperacusis, vertigo, irritability, poor concentration. Other **symptoms** are more **psychogenic** in origin and relate to previous **personality** and the psychological setting or significance of the trauma, e.g. vague physical symptoms, **anxiety, phobias.** *See also* **neurosis, compensation.**

postconcussional syndrome   The development of **symptoms** following a closed head injury, resulting in transient loss of **consciousness,** characterized by headache, dizziness, tinnitus and irritability.

posthypnotic amnesia   *See* **amnesia.**

posthypnotic suggestion   *See* **suggestion.**

postleucotomy syndrome   **Behaviour** following **leucotomy,** usually within the first few weeks, characterized by loss of social **inhibitions,** shallowness of **mood,** impulsive **behaviour, exhibitionism** and incontinence. The condition frequently improves within a month.

postpartum affective disorder   *See* **affective disorder.**

postpartum depression   *See* **depressive illness, postpartum.**

postpartum psychosis   *See* **psychosis, puerperal.**

post-traumatic amnesia   *See* **amnesia.**

post-traumatic brain syndrome   Chronic disorder following a usually severe head injury (open or closed), the nature of the **symptoms** depending partly on the site and size of the lesion but also on previous **personality.** Some symptoms, e.g. giddiness, irritability,

post-traumatic stress disorder

fatigue, **insomnia,** headache, poor concentration, excess reaction to **stress (catastrophic reaction),** are related to brain disturbances (especially located in the brain stem). Other more diffuse **neurotic** symptoms are more likely to be psychological reactions to the injury and may be related to **compensation neurosis.**

post-traumatic stress disorder *See* **neurosis, traumatic; neurosis, war.**

posturing The adoption and maintenance of extravagant or unusual bodily poses, seen in most extreme form in **catatonic schizophrenia** when a patient may lie holding his head several inches above the pillow for many hours. May also be seen in some mentally handicapped individuals.

poverty of affect *See* **affect.**

poverty of thought *See* **thought.**

Pratt, Joseph H. (b.1842) Boston physician considered the founder of **group psychotherapy**, bringing together patients with tuberculosis to benefit their morale.

precipitating aetiology *See* **aetiology.**

precipitating event External happening affecting an individual before the onset of an illness or crisis, which is believed to interact with predisposing circumstances in causing the illness. e.g. A man may discover his wife has a lover, and wander from home in a dazed state, the event having precipitated a **fugue.**

preconscious Adjective referring to **thoughts,** feelings or other information outside present awareness but readily retrievable through an act of attentive **recall.** 2. Noun referring to the class of such information. 3. In **psychoanalysis** refers to the part of the **psyche** between the **unconscious** and conscious awareness, containing thoughts, memories etc. which although not in awareness can readily become so. In contrast, the contents of the unconscious cannot become accessible to awareness through efforts at recall.

predisposition The inherited ability of an individual to develop a certain tendency or liability. The predispostion may be to develop a certain kind of illness, e.g. **schizophrenia.** *See also* **diathesis.**

pregenital In **psychoanalysis,** referring to the stages of infantile psychosocial development (**oral** and **anal**) which precede the **genital**

stage, and the impulses and **fantasies** associated with these early stages of infantile sexual life.

premenstrual tension   Behaviour occurring hours to a week before menstruation, during which the individual becomes irritable, sometimes depressed, fatigued and emotionally labile. Signs of water retention may be present or absent. The condition tends to recur on a regular basis in predisposed women, but the degree of contribution of psychological or hormonal factors is still being debated.

premonition   In the morbid sense, an intuitive awareness of future events usually with a negative connotation, e.g. doom or disaster. May occur in association with **depressive illness** or **anxiety** states.

prevalence   Frequency of a disorder. Term in **epidemiology** denoting the total number of cases per unit of population at a given time (point prevalence) or over a given period (period prevalence), e.g. one year, usually expressed as rate per 1000 population.

Prichard, J. C. (1785–1848)   British psychiatrist who described disorders of mood such as gloom or sorrow without delusions. In 1835 used the term "moral insanity" to describe intellectually normal individuals who are depraved and incapable of decency and propriety. *See* **personality disorder, sociopathic**.

primal scene   In **psychoanalysis,** the experience in childhood of witnessing sexual intercourse between the parents or, if not actually seen, the **fantasy** of having done so; related to subsequent adult psychological malfunctioning.

primary gain   Refers to the relief gained by the solution of an otherwise insoluble **conflict** by an **hysterical** illness.

primary process   In **psychoanalysis,** a primitive and often maladaptive form of mental activity characteristic of the **unconscious,** not following laws of logic or time, and guided by the **pleasure principle.** Occurs in dreaming. Mental images tend to become fused **(condensation)** and can readily replace or stand for one another **(displacement).** In **Freud's** view characteristic of infantile modes of **thought** and imagery. (cf. **Secondary process**.)

Prince, Morton (1854–1925)   American neurologist and psychiatrist who studied **multiple personality**.

prodrome   The bodily or emotional experiences immediately preceding a disease or attack of disorder, e.g. **epilepsy** or **migraine**.

projection

epileptic prodrome A disturbance of **mood** or **behaviour** (or, rarely, subjective symptoms such as headache) preceding an **epileptic seizure** by hours or days.

projection An important **defence mechanism** which consists of the attribution to others of one's own unacknowledged and undesirable **emotions,** feelings or attitudes. **Paranoid delusions** are based upon the projection of hostile or aggressive feelings.

projective test A type of psychological test aiming to determine **personality** traits through the completion of sentences, interpretation of ink blots **(Rorschach test),** interpretation of pictures **(TAT)** or the like, where the person is left to follow his own inclinations or **fantasies.**

promiscuity Sexual behaviour in which the relationship with the partner is of negligible significance, and which is relatively frequent.

prostitution The provision of a sexual partner in return for payment. Prostitutes may be either female or male. Although genital stimulation or coitus are typically involved, other types of stimulation may be provided, e.g. **sado-masochism.**

pseudocyesis False pregnancy, the woman believing wrongly that she has conceived. Occurs in **hysterical illness,** but may be a symptom of other psychiatric disorders as well. *See* **hysterical pseudocyesis.**

pseudodementia An illness with **symptoms** of impaired **memory** and intellectual functions which suggest an **organic** mental disorder but which are primarily emotional in origin. A common cause of this **syndrome** is depression, with **apathy** and impaired concentration. *See also* **Ganser state; pseudodementia, hysterical.**

depressive pseudodementia This is found in the setting of severe **depressive illness,** usually of **psychotic** or **endogenous** type in elderly subjects. A careful history will establish that the illness has begun recently and that no intellectual impairment has preceded the onset of depressive **symptoms.** The impairment in thinking appears authentic in contrast to that in **hysterical pseudodementia.** The distress of the patient is evident and there is depressive thought content which may be delusional. In severe cases incontinence of urine or faeces may heighten the resemblance to **organic dementia.** A previous history of **affective disorder** and a family history of depressive or **manic-depressive illness** is common.

hysterical pseudodementia In this disorder a whole range of **hysterical conversion symptoms** is associated with a bland, insouciant emotional attitude towards the symptoms and the traumatic or threatening situation that provoked the episode. Isolated approximate answers may be elicited but not the whole **Ganser state,** and **clouding** of **consciousness** in particular is absent. There is usually some stressful situation which has caused flight into disabling symptoms. **Brain damage** or a **neurotic** emotional disorder such as a **depressive** or **anxiety** illness may have acted to release symptoms of **hysterical neurosis.**

pseudohallucination   A subjective experience midway between imagery and **percept.** There is a lack of full external objective reality and the individual is aware of the subjective nature of the experience.

pseudologia fantastica   A tendency to elaborate extravagant **fantasies** about one's life or achievements which are presented to others as factual. A rare manifestation of **hysterical personality disorder.**

psilocybin   An indole-like substance related to **LSD,** extractable from a Mexican mushroom, which induces **hallucinations,** predominantly visual, and a transcendental **mood** in a clear **sensorium.** The clinical picture is indistinguishable from that produced by **LSD** or **mescaline.** The **drug** is used by priestesses or *curanderas* in Mexico during religious **rituals.**

psychalgia   (obs.) Pain of **psychogenic** origin. In **DSM-III,** called psychogenic pain disorder.

psychasthenia   (obs.) A condition first described by **Janet** characterized by multiple **symptoms** or oversensitivity, **anxiety** and fatigue of **psychogenic** origin. cf. **neurasthenia.**

psyche   The **mind** or the soul, as opposed to the body and the physical functioning of the person.

psychedelic   A term coined by Humphry Osmond in 1957 implying 'mind-manifesting' or capable of exerting profound effects upon the nature of conscious experience. The label is attached to **hallucinatory** or **psychotomimetic drugs** such as **mescaline, LSD** and **psilocybin** which may be categorized as major psychedelics, in contrast to the minor group which includes **cannabis** and other plant substances such as nutmeg and banana skin.

psychiatric social worker   A professional social worker who has undertaken additional training to fit him or her for **social work** with the mentally disordered.

psychiatrist A medically qualified physician who specializes in the study and treatment of mental disorders, including emotional problems, impaired relationships with others, **neuroses** and **psychoses.**

psychiatry The branch of medicine concerned with disorders of the **mind.** Thus the medical speciality dealing with the study of mental disorders, and their diagnosis, treatment and prevention.

community psychiatry The provision of mental health care to a specific population using the techniques of **epidemiology** to identify need and evaluate effectiveness, the resources of the community to support professional services, and multidisciplinary professional care outside as well as within existing psychiatric hospitals and other institutions.

descriptive psychiatry Usually denotes the aspect of clinical psychiatry concerned with **symptoms, signs** and **syndromes** of disorder as developed in the latter 19th century, e.g. by **Kraepelin.** In contrast **psychodynamic** psychiatry refers to the study of the life history, **unconscious** processes and **complexes** characteristic of the subjective life of the person, as developed by **Janet** and **Freud.** While both should be combined, in practice some psychiatrists may be adherents of one or another approach.

existential psychiatry A mode of practising psychiatry in which analysis of the patient's personal experience is paramount, and in which the individual's own capacity for finding meaning and value are explored. Based on the **existentialism** systems of philosophy of **Kierkegaard, Heidegger** and **Sartre,** as developed by **psychiatrists** such as **Binswanger** and Medard Boss.

forensic psychiatry That branch of the specialty concerned with the legal definition of insanity, with issues of **responsibility** at law of the mentally ill offender, competence to stand trial, and the operation of laws directing the disposal of the offender found incapable of issuing a plea by reason of severe **mental illness.**

geriatric psychiatry (syn. psychogeriatrics) The branch of psychiatry conerned with the diagnosis, treatment and care of mental disorder in old people.

social psychiatry The branch of psychiatry based on the applications of sociology to mental health and illness, particularly research into the effects on illness of social class, roles, deviance, community responses to the mentally ill, life stresses, hospitalization and cultural differences (transcultural psychiatry). *See also* **epidemiology psychiatry, community.**

psychic factors When used in a psychiatric context, psychic ordinarily refers to psychological or **psychogenic** aspects of an illness. In more common usage, the term refers to the excercise of occult powers.

psychoanalysis A method of treatment of the **neuroses** and other psychiatric disorders devised by **Freud** in the 1890s, and a theory about functions of the **mind,** developed subsequently by him and by his followers. The key concepts are the **unconscious** mind, the exploration of the **analysand's** mental experience through **free association** and the **interpretation** of **dreams,** often in daily sessions of about one hour extending over years. An important response of the analysand is his relationship over time with the analyst, an aspect of which is **transference.**

psychoanalytic theory Originally devised by **Freud** and refers to discrete but interrelated topics: 1. An **epigenetic** hypothesis of human psychological development through characteristic libidinal stages. 2. A structural description of the **psyche** and the constant dynamic interaction of its component entities: the **unconscious id** and **superego,** and the conscious **ego.** 3. The process and techniques of psychoanalytic **psychotherapy.** Psychoanalytic theory postulates the formative influence of early infantile experiences; the importance of infant sexuality and the **Oedipus complex;** psychic **determinism;** the dominance of unconscious **motivation** over conscious **behaviour;** the centrality of (sexual) libidinal energy; the usefulness of **dream interpretation** in therapy; the therapeutic techniques of **free association** and the analysis of **transference** and **counter-transference.** Later developments of psychoanalytic theory have modified many of the original concepts: **Jung,** an early revisionist, rejected the sexual nature of libidinal energy in favour of a universal life urge; the components of the unconscious are held by him to be archetypal figures from the common past of the race which relate to the personal experience of the individual. **Adler** added an emphasis on family birth order, the importance of the need for power, and the development of an individual lifestyle. **Anna Freud** systematically elaborated and described the mechanisms of defence against **anxiety** used by the ego. Kris, Hartmann and Lowenstein defined categories of human development (ego capacities) relatively free of unconscious **conflict. Erikson** added a social-adaptive component to the stages of epigenetic development, and a number of developmental stages to extend the description of psychic history beyond **adolescence** through early adulthood and maturity to old age. Melanie **Klein** proposed a divergent model of early infantile development, and emphasized the importance of internal objects. Kohut developed an epigenetic history of the development of the self.

psychobiology   The school of **psychiatry** developed by Adolf **Meyer,** 'the father of American psychiatry', who held that illness was to be understood by obtaining a complete history of the person, in which full account is taken of the **psychology,** the biology and the environment of the individual (1915). The related treatment approach, **distributive psychotherapy,** aims to adapt the patient to his environment by correcting faulty mental habits.

psychodrama   Devised by Moreno as a group method for the patient to act out spontaneously, with therapists and fellow actors participating, life events or formative and other crucial experiences and relationships. Usually combined with other forms of **psychotherapy.** Based on the principle that dramatic reconstruction of **conflicts,** with fellow patients helping to recreate past conflicts, has advantages over undramatized verbal communication.

psychodynamic   Pertaining to mental processes and **behaviour,** in health and disease, studied from a dynamic point of view, having regard to the interacting variables which determine emotional growth, fluctuation and change. The term generally implies an application of the principles of **psychoanalytic theory,** such as the role of **unconscious motivation.** Psychodynamic psychiatry is sometimes contrasted with **descriptive psychiatry.**

psychogenic   **Symptoms** and conditions caused by psychological factors as opposed to **organic** physical factors.

psychogenic asthma   *See* **asthma.**

psychogenic backache   Backache without detectable **organic** cause in the presence of psychological or emotional **stress.** A vague entity requiring careful physical investigation, both to find the psychological causes and to exclude physical disease.

psychogenic dermatitis   A rash due to inflammation of the skin caused by psychological or emotional factors without detectable physical cause. Associated with intense **anxiety** and **stress** in vulnerable individuals.

psychogenic dysmenorrhoea   Painful menstruation, caused by psychological or emotional factors. May be associated with excessive sexual **conflict,** poor sexual relations, difficult marriage, **premenstrual tension** and depressed **mood.**

psychogenic dyspareunia   Painful sexual intercourse caused by psychological or emotional factors. May be associated with puritanical or ambivalent attitudes to sex, poor relationship with partner, insufficient preparedness for intercourse (insufficient **foreplay**), intense **anxiety** or depressed **mood.**

psychogenic eczema Inflammatory disorder of the skin associated with itching papules and vesicles, usually associated with other atrophic features and a family history of such disorders; psychological factors contribute significantly to the course of this disorder.

psychogenic gastric ulcer An ulcer of the mucous membrane of the stomach caused by psychological **stress** in somatically predisposed individuals. Occurs most commonly on the lesser curve of the stomach. Many hypothetical factors have been implicated, e.g. the struggle between excessive dependency needs and independence, internalized self-directed **aggression.** However, specific **psychodynamic** patterns have not been well researched and remain conjectural.

psychogenic hiccough *See* **hiccough.**

psychogenic pain disorder *See* **psychalgia.**

psychogenic pruritus Itching caused by psychological factors without identifiable **organic** disorder.

psychogenic skin disorder Itching of the skin, excessive blushing, and rashes, in response to psychological factors, in the absence of identifiable **organic** cause.

psychogenic torticollis *See* **torticollis, spasmodic.**

psychogenic trauma Personal harm resulting from psychological insult, including emotional deprivation, loss of a loved person, threat, damage to self-esteem, violation of taboos etc.

psychogenic twilight state *See* **twilight state.**

psychogenic ulcerative colitis Ulceration of the mucosa and submucosa of the colon with bleeding, cramps and diarrhoea, caused or exacerbated by emotional factors such as **fear, anxiety** and **conflict.** Often described as occurring in inhibited, **obsessional** individuals relatively incapable of directly expressing **grief** and rage. Also described in conforming, easily slighted, hurt and dependent individuals. Although overactivity of the bowel is common in states of anxiety there is doubt as to whether the pathogenesis of ulcerative colitis is entirely dependent upon psychological factors.

psychogenic vomiting May occur as a **hysterical** phenomenon, usually in young women, expressing symbolically and physically some **conflict** about a notion or person. The condition is particularly difficult to manage in pregnancy, when it is said to symbolize rejection of the fetus and often is part of a complex **neurotic** state.

psychologist, clinical A graduate in **psychology** who has further training in a medical setting and undertakes treatment, assessment and research, often in the field of mental and other psychological disorders. Generally works in collaboration with **psychiatrists** or other medically qualified colleages. Usually a member of a national Psychological Association. *See* **clinical psychology**.

psychology The science devoted to the study of **behaviour,** mental processes and **personality.** Previously that branch of metaphysics concerned with mental processes.

analytical psychology The term applied to **Jung's psychoanalytic theories** and practice, with an emphasis on the personal **unconscious,** the collective unconscious which people have in common as an ancestral conferment, on archetypes (collective **symbols,** e.g. the witch, the wise old man) and on individual differences such as **introversion** versus **extraversion.**

clinical psychology The branch of applied psychology concerned with all types of patients, psychiatric, medical and surgical as regards both assessment and treatment.

dynamic psychology That psychology which includes concepts of process, **instinct** and development implying movement in contrast to those static psychologies which are more concerned with the enumeration and definition of attributes of **mind.** In practice the use of the term is largely confined to the theories underlying those **psychotherapies** derived from the work of Freud and his followers. (*See* **psychoanalysis**).

gestalt psychology Mainly a psychology of **perception** which began as a protest against reductive analysis in other contemporary systems of psychology. It developed between the European wars, in Germany and Austria, and is concerned with organized wholes or configurations, and considerations of figure versus ground. The main exponents were Max Wertheimer, Wolfgang Kohler and Kurt Koffka. Not to be confused with **Gestalt therapy.**

psychometry This is, literally, measurement in **psychology;** in practice applicable to any psychological function or trait that can be measured linearly. It is particularly applied to tests of **intelligence.**

psychomotor epilepsy *See* **epilepsy.**

psychoneurosis *See* **neurosis.**

psychopathic disorder *See* **personality disorder, sociopathic.**

psychopathology The study and description of disorders of mental functioning, with emphasis on the psychological elements in abnormal experience and on the meaning of a person's experience and exploration of his life history.

dynamic psychopathology The study of disorders in mental functioning, emphazing forces and **motivations** which give rise to abnormal **behaviour.**

psychopathy *See* **personality disorder, sociopathic.**
aggressive psychopathy *See* **personality disorder, sociopathic.**

psychopharmacology The study of **psychotropic** or psychoactive **drugs** and the effects they produce.

psychophysiological disorder A condition or **symptom** which is the adverse consequence of the effects that a mental state, e.g. **anxiety,** has on the physical state, e.g. muscle tension, some forms of physical illness (e.g. **asthma**). *See also* **psychosomatic illness.**

psychosexual disorder A **sexual disorder** in which psychological factors are believed to play a significant role. In **DSM-III** these disorders include **gender identity** disorders, paraphilias (or **sexual deviations**), dysfunctions such as **frigidity** and **impotence,** and **homosexuality. In** DSM-III homosexuality is not considered a mental disorder unless the homosexual individual finds the sexual orientation a sorce of distress.

psychosis A **mental illness** in which there is gross impairment in **reality testing,** usually evidenced by such **symptoms** as **delusions, hallucinations** or seriously disorganized **behaviour.** The individual with gross impairment in reality testing incorrectly evaluates the accuracy of his or her **perceptions** and **thoughts** and makes incorrect inferences about external reality, even in the face of contrary evidence. In lay terms psychosis encompasses insanity, madness and **lunacy.** Two forms are usually differentiated: the **organic psychoses,** when physical disease, e.g. of the brain, is present; and the **functional psychoses,** including **schizophrenia** and **manic-depressive psychosis.**

acute organic psychosis (syn. acute brain syndrome, acute **confusional state, delirium**) The acute reaction of the brain to some intra- or extracerebral disturbance. It is generally short-lived and reversible and is characterized by fluctuations (or **clouding**) of the level of **consciousness** with **confusion, disorientation, illusions** and often **hallucinations.**

psychosis

affective psychosis **Mental illness,** often recurrent, in which there is a severe disturbance of **mood** such as depression or elation, which is accompanied by one or more of the following: **delusions, perplexity,** disturbed attitude to the self, and disorder of **perception** and **behaviour;** these are all in keeping with the patient's morbid mood state. *See also* **manic-depressive illness.**

childhood psychoses A group of serious **mental illnesses** in childhood. The commonest psychosis is **early infantile autism.** Other recognized types are disintegrative psychosis associated with **organic** brain disease, and adult-type psychoses, e.g. **schizophrenia,** and **manic-depressive illness** starting in childhood.

depressive psychosis (syn. **endogenous depressive illness,** involutional **melancholia, manic-depressive psychosis,** depressed type (ICD 296.1), **manic-depressive reaction,** depressed type, **monopolar depressive illness, psychotic depressive illness).** An **affective disorder** in which the main **symptom** is pervasive depression of **mood.** Activity is often markedly reduced but there may be restlessness or **agitation.** There is a marked tendency to recurrence. Recently divided into two types: bipolar (attacks of **mania** occurring as well as depression), and unipolar (recurrent depressive psychosis or mania alone). Physical symptoms, accompanying the morbidly depressed mood, include **insomnia,** fatigue, poor appetite with weight loss, and decrease in sex drive. Feelings of **guilt** and self-reproach may be **delusional** in intensity.

epileptic psychosis Psychotic disturbances (usually of paranoid-hallucinatory type) occurring in some persons with chronic **epilepsy** (usually of **temporal lobe** origin). They may be transient and post-ictal or chronic and unrelated in time to seizures.

functional psychosis A psychosis in which no demonstrable **organic** lesion or physical abnormality can be detected in the sufferer. Includes **schizophrenia** and **manic-depressive illness.**

hysterical psychosis An acute reaction, usually with clear precipitants in which there is the sudden onset of bizarre **behaviour** that may include **delusions, depersonalization, hallucinations** and unstable **mood.** The psychosis most commonly occurs in individuals with **hysterical personality disorder** and usually resolves within a few weeks. Specific culturally distinct variants include amok, **latah,** imu, whitiko, pibloktoq (Arctic hysteria), Puerto Rican psychosis, miryachit, and olonism.

induced psychosis A form of communicable mental disorder in which a usually chronic and **paranoid psychosis,** often without florid features, develops as a result of a close relationship with another person who already has an established psychosis **(folie à**

deux). The **delusions** are at least partly shared and, rarely, several persons in close association may be affected. In **DSM-III** called shared paranoid disorder.

infective psychosis (syn. infective-exhaustive psychosis) A redundant term formerly used to describe an **acute confusional state** or **acute organic psychosis.** Acute and toxic **encephalopathy,** acute toxic **encephalitis,** acute serous encephalitis and toxic confusional state are other variants no longer in use.

Korsakoff psychosis A chronic brain disorder described by **Korsakoff** and due to thiamine deficiency commonly associated with **alcoholism.** The most striking feature is a gross **memory** defect for recent events, which the patient covers over by fabrications **(confabulation).** Other **symptoms** include **disorientation** and **confusion** in the acute stages. Characteristic neurological signs of **Wernicke's syndrome** are commonly associated with this condition.

manic psychosis Manic-depressive psychosis of manic type.

manic-depressive psychosis The term introduced by **Kraepelin** in 1896 to differentiate these psychoses from those associated with deterioration or **dementia (dementia praecox** or the group of **schizophrenias).** Included in this term are all **affective psychoses** subcategorized according to both prevailing **mood** and longitudinal pattern. Until recently **involutional melancholia** was categorized separately. **ICD-9** specifies numerous depressed and manic forms (296.0–296.6). In **DSM-III** those forms that include a history of manic episode are called **bipolar disorder.**

model psychosis An experimental psychosis induced by extreme environmental manipulation such as **perceptual deprivation,** or more commonly by **psychotomimetic drugs** such as **lysergic acid diethylamide, mescaline** or **psilocybin.**

oneiroid psychosis A **dream**-like psychotic state believed by **Mayer-Gross** (1924) to occur in individuals with a mixed schizophrenic and affective predisposition. Characterized by **clouding** of **consciousness, perplexity** and detachment from immediate external reality, it is often regarded as an acute form of **schizophrenia.** *See also* **oneirophrenia.**

organic psychosis Usually subdivided into acute, subacute or chronic. These are **syndromes** in which there is impairment of **orientation, memory,** comprehension, calculation, **learning** capacity and **judgement,** often associated with abnormality of **mood,** lowering of ethical standards, deterioration of **personality** and diminished capacity for independent decision. In all cases there is a physical basis for the disorder. *See also* **dementia; delirium.**

psychosis

paranoid psychosis A psychosis not classifiable as **schizo-phrenia** or **affective psychosis** in which **delusions** especially of being influenced, persecuted or treated in some special way are the main **symptoms.** The delusions are of a fairly fixed, elaborate and systematized kind.

post-traumatic psychosis A psychotic disorder which occurs as a late sequel of head injury. Post-traumatic **delirium, personality** changes and simple **defect states** are usually excluded. The psychosis may be a disorder of **mood** (e.g. depression), **paranoid** or **schizophreniform;** a comparatively rare consequence of **brain damage.**

puerperal psychosis Mental disorder shortly after childbirth. In the puerperium **acute psychoses** are now comparatively rare, but the risk of psychosis is lower during pregnancy and higher during the year following delivery, with the highest incidence in the first month postpartum when there is a fourfold increase in risk. Puerperal psychoses are different from those occurring at other times only by their association with major hormonal and social role changes and the fact that they are usually of acute onset and often associated with transient **clouding of consciousness. Affective disorders** are most common, often with mixed features, though pure **mania** is comparatively rare. Diagnostic confusion with **schizophrenia** is liable to occur with the florid symptomatology and **perplexity** associated with clouding of consciousness. There is no evidence that the prognosis of schizophrenia is influenced by its specific association with childbirth.

schizoaffective psychosis A psychosis in which pronounced **manic** or **depressive** features are intermingled with pronounced **schizophrenic** features, and which tends towards remission without permanent defect, but is prone to recur. The diagnosis should only be made when both the affective and schizophrenic **symptoms** are pronounced. In **DSM-III** this category does not have any specified diagnostic criteria but is to be used when a differential diagnosis between an **affective disorder** and another psychotic disorder such as **schizophrenia** cannot be made.

schizophrenic psychosis A severe **mental illness** (psychosis) with characteristic disintegration of the process of **thinking,** loss of contact with reality and emotional **withdrawal,** often with **delusions** and **hallucinations,** the severe forms resulting in progressive changes of **personality.** In 1911 **Bleuler** used the term **schizophrenia** to describe a group of disorders, previously known as

dementia praecox, in which there was a slowly progressive deterioration of the personality and characteristic disturbances of **thought, perception, mood** and **behaviour.** **Kraepelin** had divided these disorders into four categories, namely paranoid, catatonic, hebephrenic and simple. The boundaries of the concept are not well defined. Some classifications include an acute form (**ICD-9** : 295.4), whereas others (including **DSM-III**) limit the term to chronic illnesses with some signs of deterioration in functioning.

schizophreniform psychosis A **schizophrenia**-like psychosis in which there is a clear precipitating factor, relatively acute onset, a **depressive, hysterical** or **paranoid** colouring and a symptomatology which is often psychologically understandable. According to Langfeldt (1937) this condition has a benign outcome in most cases. **ICD-9** says the term should only be used as a last resort. In **DSM-III,** only distinguished from schizophrenia by its shorter duration (less than six months).

senile psychosis A progressive **senile dementia** in which senile atrophic changes in the brain are accompanied by a variety of **delusions** and **hallucinations** of a persecutory, depressive or physical nature, disturbance of **sleep** pattern and preoccupation with people or events of long ago. The preferred term is senile dementia, depressed or paranoid type (**ICD-9:290.2**).

subacute organic psychosis (subacute **confusional state ICD-9 :293.1**) Similar to **acute organic psychosis (delirium)** but usually less florid, with marked fluctuations in intensity and lasting several weeks or longer.

psychosocial dwarfism *See* **dwarfism.**

psychosomatic illness A physical illness, to which emotional factors contribute in causation, exacerbation and prolongation of the disorder. Peptic ulcer, coronary artery disease, asthma, certain skin disorders, ulcerative **colitis** and **migraine** were among the conditions thus classified. The contemporary approach is to investigate all physical illnesses for possible psychological and social components, and to regard as psychosomatic those physical illnesses found on investigation to have emotional concomitants.

psychostimulant drugs A subgroup of the stimulant group of **psychotropic drugs** which exert a direct clinical effect upon **mood,** e.g. the **amphetamines.**

psychosurgery Interruption of brain pathways or removal of regions of the brain by surgical means to alleviate psychiatric disorder.

psychotherapist A clinician who practises **psychotherapy,** in which psychological processes mediated by conversation are the main agents of treatment. The relationship between clinician and patient is of chief importance, the goal being personal development and progressive self-understanding of the patient.

psychotherapy A class of treatments based on verbal communication between patient (client) and therapist, directed at the patient's mental or emotional problems. Applicable throughout medicine, most particularly in **psychiatry** and general practice. Many types, varying in detailed aims, intensity, duration and theoretical basis, include general or **supportive,** focal or **distributive,** and formal, **interpretative** or **psychoanalytic**; special forms include **group** psychotherapy and behavioural psychotherapy.

brief psychotherapy A form of psychotherapy which focuses on goals which are expected to be achieved in 15 or 20 sessions.

distributive psychotherapy A form of psychotherapy associated with the **psychobiology** of Adolf **Meyer.** Therapy involves careful investigation of the patient's past experience, a synthesis of assets and liabilities, and efforts to devise more adaptive patterns of behaviour.

dyadic psychotherapy The psychotherapies in which two people take part, the patient and the clinician. cf. **family therapy, group therapy, psychodrama.**

group psychotherapy A form of psychotherapy applied to a group of patients, using interpersonal interactions to achieve therapeutic goals of the members of the group. More specifically a form of psychotherapy in which treatment is conducted by one or two therapists in small and carefully balanced groups (usually 6–8 persons), the members of which provide the main therapeutic potential.

interpretative psychotherapy Psychological treatment by means of a series of psychotherapeutic interviews, with the aim of changing the patient's **behaviour** and **personality** by discovering **unconscious** processes, e.g. **conflicts,** and promoting awareness of previously **dissociated** aspects of the self. The treatment approach is usually based on the theories and techniques derived from **psychoanalysis.** *See also* **interpretation.**

supportive psychotherapy The most commonly used form of psychotherapy, which provides explanation, reassurance, and advice, with the aim being to improve the patient's **adaptation.**

psychotic   Relating to **psychosis.** 2. One who is ill with psychosis; one who has lost contact with reality and is mad or insane (lay terms).

psychotomimetic drugs   Drugs which produce perceptual disturbances which may so resemble a psychosis as to be described as a model **psychosis.** *See also* **hallucinogens.**

psychotropic drugs   (syn. psychoactive drugs) Substances which act directly or indirectly upon the **central nervous system** to affect mental and emotional processes.

puberty   A stage in physical development when the reproductive system matures and secondary sexual characteristics develop. It is characterized by a variety of stages which are of variable duration and time of onset. They include spermatogenesis, onset of emissions, genital changes, pubic hair growth and voice deepening in boys; breast enlargement, genital changes, pubic hair growth and menarche in girls; and a growth spurt in both sexes. Puberty is usually earlier in girls than in boys.

puerperium, psychiatric complications   Those psychiatric conditions which follow childbirth. There is a wide variation in the literature regading the duration of the period following childbirth which should be considered, with some authorities including all disorders occurring within one year of the birth. *See also* **psychosis, puerperal.**

punch-drunkenness   **Brain damage** consisting of a traumatic **encephalopathy** occurring in boxers with **dysarthria,** cerebellar or **extrapyramidal** disturbance and occasionally asymmetrical pyramidal signs. It is virtually confined to professional boxers; most frequent in fair-booth fights, and less common since the stricter regulation by the British Boxing Board of Control.

pyknic type   A bodily configuration of roundness, with much fat tissue and large body cavities, associated with a **cyclothymic personality** characterized by cheeriness and contentment. A form of **physique.** In **Kretschmer's** system of constitutional types. *See also* **typology.**

pyromania   An old term referring to persons who repeatedly and inappropriately set fire to things. In **DSM-III,** an illness in which there is a recurrent failure to resist the impulse to set fires, and intense satisfaction in setting fires and seeing them burn.

rape A sexual assault. In legal terms means sexual (i.e. vaginal) intercourse between a man and a woman (not his wife), without the woman's consent.

rapid eye movement sleep *See* **sleep.**

rapport Harmony in communication. Applied to an individual, signifies a capacity to enter into easy emotional contact with others; applied to dyads or groups, implies shared understanding of feelings.

rationalization A term coined by Ernest Jones to mean the process of justifying or making appear reasonable an irrational or illogical act. It is a screening process intended to cover a flaw in **repression,** i.e. to cover ideas or actions which arise as gratification of an **unconscious** need. The agency is the unconscious **ego,** which evades the recognition of irrational and inconsistent **behaviour** arising on the basis of unconscious urges, e.g. a sleepless person may ascribe his **insomnia** not to **anxiety** but to heredity, saying his father slept poorly.

Raven's progressive matrices Non-verbal **intelligence test** based on appreciation of relationships of patterns.

RCBF *See* **regional cerebral blood flow.**

reaction formation A **defence mechanism** where the individual manifests attitudes and patterns of **behaviour** which are a direct antithesis to the underlying unconscious trends or impulses which continue to exist in the **unconscious.** For instance, oversolicitousness may be the conscious expression of unconscious hate. Reaction formation is a typical mechanism in **obsessive compulsive illness**.

reactive When used to describe a **mood** state refers to fluctuation with environmental change; describing a **syndrome** expresses that the syndrome developed as a result of an environmental setback.

reading disability (syn. reading disorder) A general term referring to reading difficulties in children. Often divided into reading backwardness, which refers to children backward in relation to the average attainment for their age regardless of **IQ,** and specific reading **retardation,** which refers to children whose reading difficulty is inexplicable in terms of the child's general **intelligence.** The latter may be related to **dyslexia.**

reality principle **Psychoanalytic** term; accommodation to the demands of external reality on the **psyche** characterized by logic, concern for consequences, and delay and modification of gratification. According to **Freud,** mental activity is governed by two principles, the reality principle and the **pleasure principle.**

reality testing **Psychoanalytic** term; the process of modifying **behaviour,** subjective wishes, needs, **fantasies** and **perceptions** in response to the demands of external reality. Characteristic of the mature well-integrated **psyche.**

reasoning A process of thinking, involving logical and directed sequencing of **thoughts;** inference, or the solving of problems by applying general principles.

recall The voluntary active bringing back into **consciousness** of previously stored particular memories of past events or facts learned.

receptor Specialized nerve ending capable of response to a particular class of stimulus, either from within the body or in the environment; electrical, chemical, mechanical, caloric (temperature), wave form (sound and light) etc.

recidivism A non-scientific term referring to persistent or repeated offending.

reflex Automatic, fixed, unlearned response to a stimulus not calling for conscious effort, e.g. the eye-blink reflex.

regional cerebral blood flow (RCBF) Measured by using a non-invasive technique, such as the inhalation of a safe radioactive gas (xenon 133), since blood flow is directly related to brain metabolism. Useful in charting blood flow, e.g. in differentiating pseudo-dementia from true dementia. One of the new imaging techniques. *See also* **position emission tomography.**

registrar In the field of **psychiatry** a trainee **psychiatrist,** usually in his second, third or fourth year of training. Equivalent to Resident in USA.

registration The initial phase in a **memory** process. Psychological tests of memory span measure such capacity for immediate or short-term memory.

regression Refers to the act of returning to some earlier level of psychological development or **adaptation.** Various levels or stages of development were described by **Freud** and his successors, including prenatal, infantile (including **oral, anal** and **genital stages),**

puberty, adolescence, adulthood, climacteric and senescence. Reversion to previous levels of maturity under stress or the influence of illness may be short-lived or longer-lasting. Regression is typically towards a stage, person or mode of gratification in relation to which fixation took place during development.

rehabilitation   A process of correction of the handicaps, social, psychological and physical, which arise in the wake of a disabling illness. Rehabilitation enables the patient to cope with independent existence to the extent of abilities remaining.

Reil, J. C. (1759–1815)   One of the first German physicians to devote himself to psychiatry as a specialty. Professor of Medicine at Halle and then at Berlin, he described the structure in the brain since known as the Island of Reil. He was interested in the relation between mind and body, and wrote the first systematic treatise of psychotherapy in 1803 and a detailed description of how a mental hospital should be organized. He held there are three main medical specialities: medicine, surgery and psychiatry.

reinforcement   The strengthening of a conditioned reflex in conditioning. In operant conditioning a reward is given immediately after some behaviour which is being evoked and established, e.g. a food pellet given to a laboratory animal displaying desired behaviour, and in children with autism for good behaviour. In humans, reinforcement schedules have to be individually tailored, given immediately and contingent on the behaviour being right.

relaxation   A state of repose with calmness of mind and reduced muscle tone. Systematic training to attain relaxation is a component of some forms of behaviour therapy. The state can also be promoted clinically by suggestion, hypnosis or by the use of drugs such as barbiturate administered intravenously.

reliability   Degree of dependability, trustworthiness, predictability, and freedom from observer error, e.g. of a procedure for assessing and measuring a psychological function. The reliability coefficient is the correlation between a paired series of observations made by two independently acting observers.

REM sleep   *See* sleep.

remand home   An institution which in former times received children or adolescents charged or remanded by the courts on criminal offences. Children are now committed to the care of the local authority and adolescents are committed to remand centres, or remand wings of Borstal institutions or prisons.

remembering The general term applied to the various forms of return to **consciousness** of past events or facts learned and stored in the **memory,** i.e. **recall,** recollection, recognition.

reminiscence As in general usage, it refers to a state of recalling and dwelling on memories of the past, often for long periods, in a state of lowered **attention** to the present.

repetition compulsion The impulse to re-enact earlier experiences. In **psychoanalysis** refers to the general tendency of repressed wishes or impulses to erupt into consciousness with consequent increase in **anxiety,** and activation of psychological defences against them. *See also* **undoing.**

repression The foremost of the **defence mechanisms.** The psychological process by which an idea or impulse is made **unconscious** so that the person is unaware of it. Repression results in the **personality** being in two parts. In **psychoanalysis** the repressing agency is viewed as the **superego** or **ego;** the stimulus to repression is considered to be **anxiety.** A person may repress sexual impulses regarded as objectionable, or **emotions** such as rage or hatred. The process impoverishes the self through diminishing the ego of its repressed components. *See also* **dissociation.**

reserpine An alkaloid used for treatment of hypertension and **anxiety.** It acts by depleting catecholamine stores in body tissues, including the brain. Although it was the first **drug** effective in the treatment of **schizophrenia,** it is no longer used for this purpose because of the occurrence of severe **depressive mood** in susceptible patients.

residual state An outcome of **schizophrenia;** following the **psychosis** recovery is incomplete, a **defect state** resulting, with blunting of **affect,** lack of **motivation** and traces of **hallucinations, delusions** and possibly **thought disorder.**

resistance Reluctance to face personal truths and avoidance of these by evasions and **distortions.** The use of a variety of defensive stratagems to oppose awareness of underlying motives, particularly the bringing to **consciousness** of **unconscious** processes. **Psychoanalytic** term; the conscious or unconscious defence against admitting unconscious processes, e.g. hostile or sexual impulses, into consciousness.

responsibility A legal concept referring to an individual's accountability for his actions and their consequences. An individual may be absolved from criminal responsibility by virtue of his age, or by the presence of a mental disorder which satisfies the requirements of the **McNaughton rules** or by virtue of an **automatism.**

diminished responsibility A specific defence to a charge of **murder** which is defined in section 2 of the Homicide Act, 1957. It has the effect, when successful, of reducing a charge of murder to the lesser offence of manslaughter for which the court disposal is flexible and not fixed, as it is for murder.

retardation The slowness of **thought** and/or speech found in severely depressed patients. Not to be confused with mental retardation.

reticular formation A diffuse network of neurones in the brain stem containing nuclei involved in the maintenance of **homeostasis, consciousness** and **attention.**

retirement Withdrawing into seclusion or away from contact with the world. Commonly used to mean giving up work or duty at a late stage of life. Is considered a major **stress** or transitional state, especially in men, where loss of role, status, income and occupation make demands upon the coping resources of the individual and his family.

retrograde amnesia *See* **amnesia.**

Retzustand (Ger.) *See* residual **schizophrenia, residual state.**

rigidity Unyielding, inflexible and unaccommodating attitudes or **behaviour.** 2. In **Parkinsonism,** a characteristic form of muscular stiffness when the muscles will not flex easily, **cogwheel rigidity.** 3. In the **extrapyramidal syndrome,** muscular rigidity.

cogwheel rigidity Refers to the intermittent resistance found in a limb with increased tone which is bent passively. Occurs in **Parkinsonism.**

ritual A term with various different meanings in anthropology, religion etc. In **psychiatry** it refers to patients performing repeated stereotyped series of actions, usually with pleasure and unaccompanied by the subjective sense of **compulsion.** Sometimes a private system of counter-magic to ward off imaginary fears. Seen in **schizophrenia, obsessional neurosis** etc.

Rogers, Carl R (1902–) American psychologist, best known for his system of non-directive, 'client-centred **psychotherapy**', characterized by an open, direct, 'person-to-person' relationship between the therapist and the client, 'a person of unconditional self-worth'. The therapist should be 'genuine' with **empathy** in his responses. The aim of therapy is to help the client achieve a feeling of congruence between himself and his experience, 'a situation which, if achieved, would represent freedom from internal strain and anxiety'.

role Pattern of behaviour which the person acquires and adopts in terms of what others expect of him, or which his position in the social setting assigns to him. e.g. paternal role, or as trickster in certain tribes.

role conflict Tension arising when an individual undertakes two functions which clash or compete e.g. business woman and housewife.

role diffusion Inability on the part of an adolescent to define his **identity (Erikson)**.

Rorschach, Hermann (1884–1922) Swiss psychiatrist who devised a psychological test for assessment of **personality**, using ten cards with symmetrical ink blots of varying design; the subject is asked 'what he sees on the card' and the responses can then be interpreted and scored.

Rorschach test One of the earliest and formerly widely used **projective tests,** devised by **Rorschach**. It consists of ten cards of symmetrical ink blots, some coloured, which the subject is asked to describe. An extensive scoring system and vocabulary have been devised to describe the traits delineated. The responses are held to reveal **unconscious** as well as conscious aspects of the **personality,** and to assist in the diagnosis of certain illnesses, e.g. **schizophrenia.**

rum fit *See* **fit.**

rumination Pondering repetitively for long periods on a particular problem or **thought.** The borderline between normal and abnormal is arbitrary and judged by such criteria as the trivial or unreal content of the rumination, the length of time so spent and the effectiveness or otherwise of any subsequent action on the rumination.

Rush, Benjamin (1745–1813) Wrote the first American book on mental illness, *Medical Inquiry and Observations upon the Diseases of the Mind,* 1812. Born in Philadelphia and qualified in Edinburgh. One of the signatories of the Declaration of Independence. Opposed the death penalty, ill-treatment of the insane, and slavery.

sadism

sadism A **sexual deviation** in which orgasm or other sexual gratification is obtained by inflicting torture or pain upon others. Derived from the writings of the Marquis de Sade (1740–1814). The **perversion** ranges from biting or scratching the sexual partner to physical assault or murder with mutilation of the victim's body.

sadomasochism Denotes a linked pair of sexual deviations, **sadism** and **masochism,** where sexual excitement is obtained by inflicting pain on another or by having pain or degradation inflicted on oneself.

Sakel, Manfred (1900–1957) Polish psychiatrist trained in Vienna. He introduced insulin coma therapy, the first of the shock treatments, much used for schizophrenia and now discredited. Lived in the United States in the later decades of his life.

Sartre, Jean-Paul (1905–1980) French philosopher, novellist and playwright who popularized **existentialism** as a widespread postwar intellectual movement. In *Being and Nothingness* he wrote on 'existential psychoanalysis', and spoke of bad faith as a form of deception of oneself and others characterizing an inauthentic existence.

scanning speech The tendency to produce staccato speech, often indicative of cerebellar damage.

Schilder, Paul Ferdinand (1886–1940) A Viennese physician who, in 1913, published a classic description of encephalitis periaxialis diffusa, which bears his name. After emigrating to New York, he published in 1935 *The Image and Appearance of the Human Body*, describing the **body image**. He also carried out pioneering work on child psychiatry and **group psychotherapy.**

schizoaffective disorder *See* **schizophrenia, schizoaffective.**

schizoid **Personality disorder** characterized by a group of personality traits (e.g. withdrawn, shy, shut-in, oversensitive, eccentric) first elaborated by **Kretschmer.** Said to precede the onset of **schizophrenia** in one-third of such psychoses, and to be related to **asthenic type.** The traits may exist throughout adult life without development of **psychosis.** In current US usage eccentric **behaviour** in addition to **withdrawal** usually warrants the diagnosis of schizotypal personality, rather than schizoid.

schizophrenia The group of **psychoses** characterized by **delusions,** incoherence and illogical **thinking, auditory hallucinations, passivity feelings** in which the individual experiences himself as the victim of influences that control his activities and usurp his will, and an impoverishment of his **emotions.** The **symptoms** are manifest in a state of clear **consciousness.** The result is usually a decline in performance at work, in social relationships and in personal care. The illness may be acute, or it may develop insidiously over many years, or it may recede leaving a **defect state (residual state).** The cause is still uncertain.

atypical schizophrenia An illness thought to be schizophrenic which does not fit comfortably into one of the established subcategories.

catatonic type schizophrenia Psychomotor disturbances are prominent, e.g. **hyperkinesis, stupor, automatic obedience, negativism, flexibilitas cerea** (semi-rigid maintained postures).

disorganised type schizophrenia *See* **schizophrenia, hebephrenic.**

hebephrenic schizophrenia A schizophrenic syndrome characterized by shallow and inappropriate **affect, thought disorder** and unpredictable **behaviour.** In the United States now called disorganized type schizophrenia.

latent schizophrenia A condition where inconsequential **behaviour** or eccentric manner may develop together with disturbances of **affect** which have a schizophrenic flavour, though no very definite signs of the illness can be elicited. *See also* **borderline state.**

nuclear schizophrenia A **psychotic** illness with **thought disorder** and disturbance of **perception, mood** and **behaviour,** where the first rank **symptoms** of schizophrenia are unequivocally present. There is often an associated deterioration of **personality.**

paranoid schizophrenia A form characterized by the predominance of **delusions,** often of a **paranoid** nature, and **hallucinations.**

paraphrenic schizophrenia *See* **paraphrenia.**

process schizophrenia (syn. nuclear schizophrenia) A schizophrenic illness with poor outcome, with first rank **symptoms** (described by **Schneider**) of schizophrenia, a high risk of deterioration and low probability of complete remission.

pseudoneurotic schizophrenia *See* **borderline state.**

residual schizophrenia A chronic **residual state** following recovery from a more severe schizophrenic episode. Although fragments of **hallucinations** and **delusions** may persist, **psychotic symptoms** are no longer prominent. The disorder is characterized by poverty of **motivation,** blunting of **affect,** and social **withdrawal.** *See also* **defect state.**

schizoaffective schizophrenia There is intermingling of **manic** or **depressive symptoms** with schizophrenic features and a tendency towards remission without **personality** defect. In the United States this condition is now considered a separate disorder rather than a subtype of schizophrenia.

schizophrenia simplex Outmoded term for schizophrenic illness with gradual onset of eccentricity, social incompetence and self-absorption. Other prominent schizophrenic features are not found.

schizophrenic episode A bout of schizophrenic illness occurring for the first time or as a recurrence, either with intervening normality or as an exacerbation of a chronic state.

schizophrenic residual state *See* **schizophrenia, residual.**

Schnauzkrampf (Ger) A stereotyped pursing or screwing up of the lips, usually associated with other **mannerisms,** especially of the face. First described as a feature of catatonic **schizophrenia,** but is also said to be a feature of the extrapyramidal side-effects of the **neuroleptics** in the sometimes irreversible **syndrome** of **tardive dyskinesia.**

Schneider, Kurt (1887–1967) German psychiatrist who made extensive contributions to the field of clinical **psychopathology,** especially from the standpoint of **phenomenology**, and also to the study of psychopathic **personality**. He proposed 'first rank' **symptoms** for the diagnosis of **schizophrenia.**

school refusal (syn. school phobia) A **fear** of going to school or, more appropriately, fear of leaving home. A common childhood disturbance which may occur during the early school years, but most often begins at the age of 11 or 12. To be distinguished sharply from **truancy**. Often arises out of separation anxiety.

scoptophilia Pleasure in looking; another term for **voyeurism.**

screen memory *See* **memory.**

secondary gain Refers to psychological benefits which accrue additionally from an illness. More specifically refers to the employment of a **hysterical** mechanism to solve **conflict**. (cf. **primary gain**)

secondary process In **psychoanalysis,** mental functioning governed by the laws of grammar, logic and time, serving the **reality principle** by adaptive **behaviour.** Developed with the **ego** as the child matures, and is associated with verbal thinking. Immediate gratifications are governed by considerations of safety, social expectations and future rewards. (cf. **primary process**).

sedatives **Drugs** which produce a calming or soothing effect, promoting rest or **sleep.** The distinction between sedatives and **hypnotics** is largely a question of dosage since small doses of hypnotics produce sedation. **Tranquillizers** are distinguished from the traditional sedative by the fact that large (hypnotic) doses of sedatives produce deep sleep or **coma,** whereas there is little or no drowsiness after large doses of a tranquilliser.

self-inflicted poisoning Alternative term for attempted **suicide** (or parasuicide or deliberate self-harm) by **drug** overdosage.

self-mutilation Many **cultures** require bodily mutilations, especially as part of **puberty** rites that may appear bizarre or cruel to members of other societies. However, some patients, usually **schizophrenics,** or the severely subnormal, may mutilate their own bodies in ways not thus accepted (e.g. castration). Minor hurts to one's own body often occur that on study turn out to have been motivated in a self-punishing way or to relieve **tension.** Only some are connected with suicidal intent; more often they are in the nature of attention-seeking gestures (wrist-slashing especially). Disturbed adolescents may inflict numerous superficial incisions on their arms or other parts of their bodies as attention-seeking or tension-relieving manoeuvres. The last are much commoner in women than in men and may reach epidemic proportions in some closed groups.

senescence Growing old.

senile Pertaining to or characterizing old age; usually implying serious deterioration or disintegration. *See also* **dementia; psychosis.**

senium The period of life after the age of 65 years.

sensitiver Beziehungswahn (Ger. lit. sensitive **delusions of reference**) The paranoid development of the shy introverted **personality** who tends to believe that others know and laugh about, for example, his or her sexual needs, or his or her masturbatory **behaviour.** They feel shamed, laughed at, perplexed and rejected, and are unable to form ordinary human relations and are prone to develop a **paranoid psychosis.**

sensorium Those aspects of **consciousness** concerned with **perception** of all the sensory experiences. In psychiatric practice, the examination of the sensorium means asking about the quality of the special sense perceptions. Clear sensorium is equivalent to full consciousness.

sensory deprivation *See* **deprivation, perceptual.**

separation anxiety Psychological **symptoms** of wide variety and usually in childhood, directly attributable to separation from another close person, most often a parent figure. *See also* **attachment.**

serotonin (5-Hydroxytryptamine, 5-HT) In the brain, a chemical **neurotransmitter** concerned with the regulation of **mood, sleep,** pain and temperature.

sex chromosome *See* **chromosome.**

sex chromosome anomalies Anomalies of the number of sex chromosomes that result from non-disjunction producing a monosomy (45X, **Turner's syndrome**) or trisomies, e.g. 47 XXY (**Klinefelter's syndrome**), 47 XYY or 47 XXX. If non-disjunction occurs during early mitosis, mosaics may result, i.e. mixture of normal and aneuploid cells. *See also* **chromosomal sex; chromosome; chromosome anomalies.**

sexual deviation (syn. **perversion, psychosexual disorder**) Sexual activity deviating from the normal. Habitual sexual act which is not heterosexual intercourse, but instead exciting erotic thoughts or **orgasm** in connection with non-consenting partners, or with animals or things, or involving debasement or suffering. Includes **homosexuality, bestiality, fetishism, exhibitionism, sadism, masochism** etc. More common in men than in women, and sometimes an accompaniment of psychiatric illness.

sexual disorders A chronic problem mainly derived from an individual's sexual preferences, responses or relationships.

sexual identity Maleness or femaleness as determined biologically by the genetic constitution, hormone secretion and genital anatomy. *See also* **gender identity.**

sexual unresponsiveness *See* **frigidity; impotence.**

shadow *See* **Jung.**

shared paranoid disorder *See* **psychosis, induced.**

shell shock A now obsolete term in general use in or after the 1914–1918 war with reference to multiple, mainly psychological, **symptoms** affecting combat soldiers who had apparently suffered no **organic** injury to account for them.

sibling   Strictly one of two or more children, not simultaneously born, of the same two parents. The term, however is often used more loosely to mean brothers and sisters, and to include twins, half-brothers and half-sisters and step-brothers and step-sisters.

sibling rivalry   The intense and emotional competition between **siblings** for the affection, approval, attention and love of one or both parents. This can be an important determinant of later character traits, and can find expression in personal relationships outside the family.

side effects   All drugs and physical methods of treatment will depend upon a main chemical or physiological action for the therapeutic benefit. The majority of such treatments will have subsidiary actions not essential for benefit but which will be powerful enough to produce an alteration in the patient's feeling of well-being. These subsidiary effects may add to the patient's distress, and may at times make the treatment burdensome. Much activity is currently taking place within the pharmaceutical industry to produce psychotropic drugs with fewer side effects.

sign   An objective manifestation (e.g. dilated pupil, absent knee jerk, rash) indicating the presence of illness that is evident to the doctor, but often not apparent to the patient. cf. **symptom.**

significant life event   Major change in the life of an individual that may adversely affect his or her health. Any happening (e.g. **bereavement,** moving house etc.) to a person, which may be accurately described and rated as regards its stressfulness by standardized techniques. The main research use is the relation of such events to the precipitation (or relief) of illness episodes, whether medical or psychiatric, e.g. the relation of bereavement to **depressive illness.**

situational disturbance   Any acute mild psychiatric disorder reactive to a particular environmental **stress.**

Skinner, Burrhus Fredeni (1904–)   Harvard psychologist whose *The Behaviour of Organisms*, published in 1938, and *Science and Human Behaviour*, published in 1953, laid the foundations of postwar behavioural **psychology**. His novel *Walden Two* describes a Skinnerian behaviourist Utopia. He has made notable contributions in two important fields, **learning theory** and **conditioning.**

sleep   A recurrent healthy state, usually occurring in a regular way at night, of unresponsiveness and inertia, with **consciousness** lost and

sleep rhythm inversion

the electrical brain waves changing in character.

paradoxical sleep A now little used term for **rapid eye movement** (REM) **sleep.**

rapid eye movement (REM) sleep A stage of sleep with rapid, conjugate movements of the eyes, accompanied by typical **EEG** changes, autonomic arousal and muscular relaxation. REM episodes occur at intervals of 70–90 minutes and may be affected by mental disorders and **hypnotic drugs. Dreams** are more commonly reported following REM periods than in other stages of sleep.

sleep rhythm inversion A rare condition of wakefulness at night and sleepiness by day, typically due to virus infections of the **central nervous system**, especially **encephalitis.**

slip of the tongue *See* **parapraxis.**

social class Categorization of individuals in a population, usually in terms of occupation of the householder or socio-economic position. In Great Britain five classes are recognized from professional (I) to unskilled labouring (V). Certain disorders are found to occur more often (allegedly) among the affluent (e.g. **anorexia nervosa),** others among the poorly off (e.g. **schizophrenia, sociopathy).** Psychiatric treatment is also associated with social class, intensive **psychotherapy** or **psychoanalysis** being prescribed more often for Class I and **electroconvulsive therapy** for Class V. *See also* **social drift.**

social drift The movement of individuals from one social category to another, sometimes as a result of morbid processes.

social isolation A physical or psychological distancing of an individual from others for whatever reason. Occurs, for example, with **schizoid personality disorder, schizophrenia, paranoid illness.**

social psychiatry *See* **psychiatry.**

social work The deployment of particular professional skills designed to assist the individual in his social adjustment. Done by a social worker employed by a local authority or hospital or other agency. One of the helping professions. *See also* **psychiatric social worker.**

sociopathic disorder *See* **personality disorder, sociopathic.**

sociopathy *See* **personality disorder, sociopathic.**

sodomy An 'unnatural' form of sexual intercourse; usually refers to anal intercourse. *See also* **paederast.**

solvent abuse   The inhalation of volatile solvents has a long history, but in recent years is said to be most common in native peoples undergoing cultural change. It occurs where access to other intoxicants is limited by confinement or economic factors, but currently it is endemic among young people in urban areas where glues are most popular. **Intoxication** and other **distortions** of **consciousness** are the main effects. *See also* **glue sniffing; petrol sniffing.**

somnambulism   (*syn.* noctambulism) Sleep-walking, occasional episodes of which may occur in otherwise normal children. If persistent, especially in adults, it is usually a sign of psychological **stress.** Those affected rarely injure themselves, and in some cases there may be a **dissociation** of waking **consciousness** rather than true **sleep.**

somnolence   In normal persons an inclination to **sleep** which occurs with boredom or lack of sleep etc. but occasionally, especially if prolonged, it may be due to chronic **drug** overdosage, toxic conditions affecting the **central nervous system,** cerebral tumour or many other conditions.

speech disorders   Difficulties in the production of spoken language, as distinct from problems of recalling words and conceptualizing language. These two areas of difficulty are not always easily distinguished, especially in the mentally handicapped and deaf where **learning** to articulate is incomplete. Nevertheless **stammering,** difficulties in articulation, and **dysarthria** from muscular and more peripheral nerve damage, as well as cerebellar disorders and various forms of functional misarticulation are usually covered by this expression. *See also* **scanning speech.**

spina bifida   A congenital deformity of the spine, leaving neural tissue exposed at the small of the back. Very mild cases may be **symptom**-free; as severity increases malfunction of bowel and bladder control and lower limb paralysis appear, and very severe cases are incompatible with life. Without early operation, damage progresses, and operation cannot correct existing damage to function. The cause of the condition is unknown, but vitamin deficiency in the diet of the pregnant mother has been suggested.

Spitz, René A. (1887–1974)   Born in Vienna, he worked there initially and then in various parts of Europe and the United States. After early collaboration with Sandor Ferenczi he returned to Vienna to be analysed by **Freud** in 1910–11, in what has been described as the first training analysis. Later became a pioneer of direct observation and photography as a means of studying infant–mother interactions. His major work was concerned with the psychic development of infants and young children. He described **anaclitic** depression (1946) in infants separated from their mothers.

splitting   A mental process (**defence mechanism**) by which the mind loses its integration and is thereby divided into two or more components such as a good self and a bad self. Parts of the self can be disowned (**repression**) or attributed to others (**projections**).

stammering   An impediment in speaking in which the normal flow of words is interupted by involuntary blocks, repetition or prolongation of sounds. A disorder of childhood, which often improves spontaneously or with **speech therapy.** Becomes more exaggerated under conditions of emotional **stress.** Not associated, as often believed, with **left-handedness.** Not a **symptom** of any physical disease. *See also* **stuttering.**

Stekel, Wilhelm (1868–1940)   Viennese **psychoanalyst** whose paper on early sexual experiences of children was quoted by **Freud.** Prolific sometimes superficial writer. Responsible for the term **thanatos** for the death wish.

Stengel, Erwin (1902–1973)   British, formerly Viennese, psychiatrist working latterly in London and Sheffield, who studied **suicide** and attempted suicide and the classification of mental disorders.

stereotyped activities   In certain mental states, especially **obsessional neurosis** and **schizophrenia,** activities are initiated which tend to be repeated. These constant and repeated activities are so-called stereotyped activities.

stereotypies   The repeated gestures, phrases or movements which are often fragmented and do not add to the intended verbal communication, but which may have a cryptic symbolic meaning for the individual, who may be schizophrenic, demented, mentally retarded, have had **encephalitis** or **Parkinsonism,** or merely be an awkward and sensitive person.

stigma   Social disgrace or rejection. A mark or lesion on the skin.

stigmata   Marks resembling the wounds of Christ's crucified body, most commonly reported in women.

stimulants   **Drugs** increasing the activity of certain organs or functions. In the case of the brain, usually refers to those increasing the level of alertness and **motivation.** (e.g. **amphetamine,** caffeine)

strephosymbolia   An old term for specific **reading disability** applied particularly to those children who reverse letters (e.g. b for d).

stress   An interference or change in conditions affecting the individual which has an adverse effect, such as worry or hostility especially when prolonged; also external conditions producing **anxiety,** as in armed combat. When protracted it can lead to physical illness. *See also* **psychosomatic disorder.**

stupor   An abormal state of absence of voluntary activity, movement, or expression of **emotion,** in either clear **consciousness** or near unconsciousness. Occasionally used to include **organic** states such as frontal lobe or other **brain tumors,** in which there is usually some **clouding** of consciousness. Stupor occurs in **catatonic schizophrenia, mania** and **depressive illness.**

Sturge-Weber syndrome   A knot of distended blood vessels on the surface of the brain, compressing it from birth, associated with a purple birthmark on the face. The underlying brain is often calcified, and common **symptoms** are **epilepsy,** hemiplegia and mental subnormality.

stuttering   The impediment in speaking in which the beginnings of words, in particular, are rapidly repeated. *See also* **stammering.**

sublimation   A socially acceptable substitute activity which provides some measure of gratification to an instinctual impulse which is unacceptable in its original form. This is not a true **defence mechanism** since it does not lead to any restriction or inhibition of **ego** function. e.g. Latent **paedophilia** in the case of some youth leaders.

subnormality   *See* **mental retardation.**

suggestibility   The extent to which an individual will accept, and act upon, ideas provided by others. A **personality** trait, increased in certain illnesses such as **hysterical conversion neurosis, catatonic schizophrenia,** and as evidenced by a hypnotized person.

suggestion   The process whereby an individual is presented with ideas in a way which facilitates their acceptance. Depends on a person's submissiveness and uncritical acceptance of influence brought to bear by, for example, a hypnotist or other persuader.

post-hypnotic suggestion   Subjects under **hypnosis** can be given orders to carry out actions after the period of hypnosis has been terminated. Many such actions may be inexplicable to the subjects

suicide

when they perform them, but it has not been proved that they can be induced to carry out actions contrary to their moral code (e.g. violence).

suicide The act of killing oneself. This is frequently, though not invariably preceded by serious mental disorder.

suicide attempt Deliberate self-harm not resulting in **death.** May be difficult to evaluate in any one case the extent to which a true self-destructive wish was operating.

hanging in suicide Commoner in male than in female suicides. Apparent suicide by hanging may occasionally be masochistic exercises which have gone wrong. This rare event is most likely to occur in teenagers and young adults.

Sullivan, Harry Stack (1892–1949) American psychiatrist generally grouped with the **neo-Freudian** psychoanalysts. His central concern was with interpersonal relations, and the effect of socio-cultural factors on development. His principal concepts are that man is an inescapably social being with specific human characteristics. Personality, a 'self-system', develops through the mirroring activity of significant others. Anxiety, the prime **motivation** of **behaviour** is engendered by social contact; at first with the mother and later with others. 'Dynamisms', integrated complexes of psychological and physical behaviour, are directed at reducing anxiety. Successful coping with anxiety is 'integrative', and unsuccessful coping produces 'disintegration'. **Mental illness** and emotional disturbances result from lack of self-esteem. Interpersonal communication is a vital psychiatric concern: 'Prototaxic' communication is the most disordered, representing discontinuity between the self and the outside world; parataxic communication is distorted; 'syntaxic' communication is the mature mode of shared, appropriate communication, in which "consensual validation", the affirmation of the self and its percepts, occurs. Sullivan did not subscribe to Freud's stages of development. Sexuality is to be regarded as but one of many needs. Sullivan was particularly innovative in the psychotherapeutic and hospital treatment of schizophrenia, in which he emphasized the learning of correct patterns of interpersonal communication and behaviour.

superego In **psychoanalysis,** the **unconscious** part of the **mind** reflecting parental prohibitions and demands, as incorporated in childhood, and hence in conflict with the **ego.** Constitutes a self-critical, self-attacking inner agency, experienced consciously as self-reproach, **guilt** or **unworthiness.** Not the same as the **conscience.** With the ego, in conflict against the amoral forces of the **id.**

superstition An irrational **belief** in chance, magic, harm in innocuous occurrences or portents. Differs from a **delusion** in that it will be found to occur in common with others in the same society who are also not ill.

surrogate One who takes the place of another. Surrogate parenting through fostering or adoption is now commonly used in providing care for deprived children. To some degree relationships, in childhood and **adolescence** particularly, may be understood in terms of surrogate-seeking usually for one or other parent. In the context of sex therapy, sexual dysfunction particualrly in the male may be treated using a surrogate partner.

symbiosis A relationship of interdependence between closely associated persons who thereby forfeit their autonomy and, if mentally disturbed, reinforce each other's **psychopathology**.

symbol A material, objective representation of a repressed object or action. A symbol represents something else (its referent). In **psychoanalytic theory,** a symbol is a representation by substitution or displacement of an object or activity that is repressed. In contrast, universal symbols (in **dreams,** mythology and folklore) refer to the perennial interests of mankind, e.g. the judgemental father, the comforting mother, the redeeming child etc.

symptom A subjective **percept** of illness, i.e. an indication of ill-health directly observed by the patient or those in his environment. The presence of disease is inferred from symptoms (and **signs**).

synaesthesia Stimulation of one sensory modality producing a response in a different sensory modality, e.g. striking an object to produce a sound will elicit a visual response of flashing coloured lights in synchrony with the sound. This phenomenon is frequently observed after ingestion of **hallucinogens.** *See also* **lysergic acid diethylamide.**

syncope Transient loss of **consciousness** due to reduction in cerebral blood flow. This can follow **emotion,** sudden changes in posture, prolonged standing, especially in the heat, and following a heavy meal, violent coughing, pressure on the neck and even, for unknown reasons, micturition. Syncope can also follow paroxysmal tachycardia and more serious heart, lung and vascular diseases.

syndrome A set of **symptoms** occurring together regularly and thus constituting a distinct clinical entity indicative of a disease or illness. Often named after the physician who first observed the condition in a group of patients, e.g. **Down's syndrome** (mongolism).

syphilis   The pathological process resulting from venereal infection by the spirochaete *Treponema pallidum*. The primary stage refers to local evidence of infection, 'the chancre', and the secondary to a process of dissemination of the spirochaete throughout the body. *See* **neurosyphilis** for the tertiary stage.

Szasz, Thomas S. (1920–)   Contemporary American psychiatrist who has written extensively (e.g. (*The Myth of Mental Illness*) questioning the validity of the concept of **mental illness**. *See also* **Laing** (antipsychiatry).

T-group   A sensitivity training group based upon **psychodynamic** (especially Bion) and educational principles. There are regular meetings with a specified leader, and the tasks of the participants include learning about themselves, interpersonal relationships, group processes and larger social systems through actual experience within the group.

taboo   Prohibitions and restrictions interwoven in the **culture**. An object is taboo if it is untouchable; an act is taboo if it is forbidden by the society. In **psychoanalysis,** therefore, there is emphasis on an incest taboo.

tactile agnosia   *See* **agnosia.**

tardive dyskinesia   Stereotyped movements of the tongue and face, often repetitive chewing, sometimes extending to movements of the body and limbs, and believed to result from the effect, at times, of **neuroleptic** drugs on the brain. A complication of long-term medication in chronic psychiatric illness.

TAT   *See* **Thematic Apperception Test.**

Tay-Sachs disease   A degenerative disease of the **central nervous system** due to disorders of lipid storage. A hereditary condition due to a **recessive gene** 100 times more prevalent in Ashkenazi Jews than in others. There are three types recognized, depending on the hexosaminidase isoenzyme defect. After a few months the newborn develops very slowly, may have **convulsions** and eventually becomes blind, developing a characteristic cherry-red spot in the macular region of the eye. The head enlarges and the child dies due to feeding and respiratory difficulties and infections. Treatments are ineffectual.

teeth grinding (bruxism) The rhythmic or spasmodic grinding or gnashing of the teeth, which may cause extreme wear of the occlusive surfaces. It is common during **sleep,** but more extreme forms are commonly associated with tension or dental malocclusion. Rarely, it occurs in **anorexia nervosa** or the **dietary chaos syndrome,** as if as an alternative to chewing food.

telepathy The unproven ability to receive feelings or information from another person without the use of the usual sensory channels.

temporal lobe epilepsy *See* **epilepsy.**

tension headache Headache seemingly related to psychological **stress** and tension and sometimes thought to be of a specific character (e.g. tight band around the head).

testamentary capacity The capacity of an individual to understand the nature and extent of his estate and those who have claims upon his bounty. To have 'a sound disposing mind' a person must have a true appreciation of his financial worth and be able to identify those who through ties of family or friendship might have reasonable claims upon him, and to formulate a clear and coherent statement regarding the disposal of his estate. An individual suffering from severe mental disorder may none the less at the time of making a will be fully competent, and it is incumbent upon a medical adviser present at the time to make and keep careful notes of the patient's mental and physical state.

thanatology The study of **death** and **dying** with emphasis on therapeutic interventions with the dying and their survivors.

thanatomania (obs.) Homicidal or suicidal **mania.**

thanatophobia Morbid **fear** of **death.**

thanatos The Greek word for **death** used by Freud (1921) in *Beyond the Pleasure Principle* to represent the **death instinct** as the dominant biological drive.

thematic apperception test (TAT) A projective test invented by Henry A. Murray at Harvard in the 1930s, and consisting of cards showing vaguely outlined human figures in various groupings on the basis of which the subject is encouraged to make up a story.

therapeutic community An institution, often psychiatric, which provides a living-learning situation through group processes emphasising social, environmental and personal interactions which are the primary mode of therapy. Self-determination, trust, respect and management by group consensus contrast with the more usual hierarchical organization of therapeutic services.

thinking   Working out in the **mind**. A sequence of ideas initiated by a problem. Mental activity involving symbols.

distorted thinking   A pattern of **thought** in which the connections between thoughts are abnormal, and the significance given to events is unusual or idiosyncratic.

magical thinking   A form of **reasoning** present in all children until the age of seven, described by **Piaget.** Psychological rather than objective explanations are used for events. Inanimate objects are endowed with feelings and intentions. Explanations are not deduced from observations, and argument is not based on facts. Persists in adulthood when a childlike view of events is taken on the omnipotent expectation that an outcome will result from personal actions rather than from a real occurrence.

thought   The act of **thinking.**

autistic thought   A pattern of **thinking** which indicates self-absorption to the exclusion of most social or external experience.

thought blocking   A **symptom** of **schizophrenia,** where there is the conscious experience of thought suddenly ending for a period, which may be observed as an unexpected and unexplained interruption of speech.

incoherence of thought   A thought process where successive concepts in the sequence of thinking bear little relation to each other.

poverty of thought   An observed lack of spontaneous ideas suggesting a dullness and lack of conceptual linking in the mental life.

tangential thought   The observation of deviation from a line of argument, taking its origin from one step of the argument, but rapidly becoming totally irrelevant.

thought disorder   A collective term for evidence of abnormal thinking processes consistent with the presence of a **psychotic** illness, particularly **schizophrenia.**

thumb sucking   The earliest manipulation of the body to develop. It may occur in the newborn, is not uncommon in babies, and occurs in most children at some time. Unlike **nail biting,** which is associated with tension, thumb sucking although associated with hunger in the first months of life is usually a source of pleasure or comfort. It becomes a problem only if accessory movements, local damage to teeth, lips or jaws develop, or if it is a source of social embarrassment.

thyrotoxicosis *See* **hyperthyroidism.**

tics Frequently repeated, abrupt, short-duration movements of muscles or muscle groups which are not under voluntary control but are usually the result of embarrassment or other **emotions.** They disappear in **sleep.** They are more common in boys and also in early life, often disappearing after months or years. Sometimes the condition is of organic origin following **encephalitis** or **cerebral degeneration.** They can be associated with compulsive swearing in, for example, the **Gilles de la Tourette syndrome,** which, like related syndromes, seems to be partly genetic in origin.

tobacco dependence Physical and psychological **dependence** on the active ingredient of tobacco, i.e. nicotine, and on the smoking habit.

token economy A means of shaping the **behaviour** of chronic **psychotic** or mentally handicapped patients in a more socially acceptable direction by the systematic rewarding of a desired behaviour by giving tokens on an overtly defined scale. The tokens can later be exchanged for privileges. *See also* **behaviour therapy.**

tolerance Occurs when, as a result of repeated prior use of a **drug,** the usual effects can only be produced by taking a higher dose.

cross tolerance Where repeated or continuous administration of a **drug** has induced **tolerance** there may be cross tolerance to the effects of pharmacologically related drugs so that the dosage of these drugs must be increased to obtain an expected therapeutic effect.

tomboyishness Style of **behaviour** in certain prepubertal girls associated with interests, preferences and pursuits generally regarded as more appropriate for boys of a similar age.

tomography *See* **computerized axial tomography.**

torticollis A condition produced by spasm of the neck muscles which may be intermittent or continuous, leading to a sideways posture of the head and eventual deformity of the neck. It is often resistant to treatment.

spasmodic torticollis Essentially a condition of adult life twice as common in women, in which a **tic**-like or tonic or clonic contraction of the neck muscles occurs pulling the head to one side. The origin is disputed and while **psychogenic** factors often seem to be very obvious, psychiatric treatments are disappointing.

toxic effect   The effect of a **drug** which is damaging to the body due to an additional pharmacological action or sensitivity, often not suspected, and which does not relate to the drug's primary mode of action, e.g. **Parkinsonism** with **phenothiazines,** dryness of the mouth with **antidepressant drugs.**

trance   A dazed state with reduced response to events and stimuli, common in **hysterical** illness, ecstatic conditions, in association with certain forms of **epilepsy,** etc.

> **hysterical trance**   A state of **dissociation** characterized by lack of voluntary movement and often by **automatisms** in act and **thought.** Occurs also in **hypnosis** and under the influence of a medium or primitive healer, shaman, **voodoo** practitioner etc.

tranquillizers   **Drugs** used in the treatment of some types of **mental illness,** or for controlling disturbed **behaviour,** by reducing **anxiety** or **agitation** and inducing a serene or placid state. Selective in action (cf. **sedatives),** intended to avoid causing **somnolence.** Major tranquillizers are now usually categorized as **neuroleptics,** and minor tranquillizers (such as the **benzodiazepines)** as **anxiolytics.**

transactional analysis   A form of **psychotherapy** devised by Eric Berne in which the **behaviour** of the patient or client is explored by studying his transactions with other people as expressions of his component inner ego states (child, parent and adult).

transference   The process whereby positive or negative **emotions** experienced during an early stage of psychological development shift from their original target to become focused upon a person or object important in the individual's later experience. The process may help or hinder medical and psychiatric treatment, and the patient's transference relationship with the clinician is a necessary component of **interpretative psychotherapy.**

translocation   *See* **chromosome anomalies**.

trans-sexualism   A disorder in which there is a persistent sense of discomfort and inappropriateness about one's anatomical sex and a persistent wish to be rid of one's genitals and to live as a member of the other sex. A man believes himself to be or wants himself to be accepted as a woman, or conversely a woman as a man. Typically a trans-sexual person seeks sex reassignment surgery to make his or her body more consistent with the preferred **gender identity.**

transvestism   The condition of wearing clothing of the opposite sex. In heterosexual men recurrent and persistent **cross dressing** may occur without overt sexual association. When for the purpose of sexual excitement, associated with **masturbation** and other sexual **behaviour** it is a form of **fetishism.** To be distinguished from **trans-sexualism,** e.g. when the cross dressing is an expression of **gender identity** disorder.

tremor A rhythmical alternating movement or shaking of the head, tongue or one or more limbs, usually involuntary, that may be fine or coarse, fast or slow, regular or irregular. There are numerous causes, medical, neurological and psychiatric, their differentiation depending as much on associated physical **signs** and **symptoms** as on analysis of the tremor. *See also* **tremor, hysterical.**

hysterical tremor May be a fine tremor resembling a state of extreme **fear** or a coarse shaking intensified by voluntary movement. It is irregular, variable and is increased when **attention** is directed to it and diminished when attention is distracted.

trichotillomania A morbid habit of twisting, plucking or pulling the hair, which may extend to pulling out hair from the head, pubic area, eyelids etc. in a compulsive way. A **symptom** of psychological tension, it is a form of **self-mutilation.** Seen in young girls most often, and in mental defect.

tricyclic antidepressant drugs A range of **antidepressant drugs** first introduced in the late 1950s, effective in the treatment of **depressive illness.** The therapeutic effect is believed to be related to the potentiation of **amines** in the **brain.** Includes amitriptyline (Tryptizol), imipramine (Tofranil), trimipramine (Surmontil) etc. Side-effects include drowsiness, dry mouth, blurred vision and **tremor** of the hands, and do not necessarily imply that medication must be stopped.

trisomy *See* **chromosome anomalies.**

truancy Deliberate evasion of attending school, the child usually not being at home either in contrast to **school refusal.**

Tuke, William (1732–1822) English Quaker philanthropist who with the Society of Friends founded the York Retreat to provide institutional care for the mentally ill which was humane.

tuberous sclerosis *See* **epiloia.**

Turner's syndrome *See* **XO syndrome.**

twilight state Partial disturbance of **consciousness.** It can be caused by a variety of conditions, e.g. after epileptic attacks, in other **organic confusional states,** in **alcoholism.** Acts may be performed which the person has not consciously willed, about which he is afterwards partly or wholly unaware. Commonly lasts for a few hours.

epileptic twilight state A condition of disturbed **consciousness** in which some normal activities are carried out, but with impaired awareness and loss of **memory** afterwards, lasting usually for a few hours after an epileptic attack.

psychogenic twilight state A state of **clouding** of consciousness which occurs in profoundly disturbed emotional states; clearly related to **hysterical trance** states but must be carefully observed so as to exclude **organic** causes.

twin research A powerful method of investigating the relative importance of **genetic** and environmental factors in illness causation. Systematic comparisons are made of the concordance of morbidity in identical and non-identical twins. A refinement of the method involves a study of twins brought up apart.

typology An approach to the study of **personality** by attempting to classify individuals as being of a certain type. Hippocrates related psychological types to 'bodily humours' (blood, phlegm, black bile and yellow bile), and Sheldon to body build, i.e. endomorph, mesomorph and ectomorph, corresponding to **Kretschmer's pyknic,** athletic and leptosomatic types.

tyramine S-Hydroxyphenylethylamine, a constituent of many foods such as beans, marmite, cheese, wine etc., which is metabolized quickly in the body by oxidation by monoamine oxidases and which has noradrenaline-like actions of raising the blood pressure, increasing the heart's stroke volume, leading to uterine and bronchial constriction, and raising the blood sugar. Responsible for the hypertensive reaction to such foods and certain drugs in patients taking a **monoamine oxidase inhibitor drug;** the rise induced in blood pressure by tyramine can lead to subdural haemorrhages and **death.**

uncinate fit *See* **fit.**

unconscious Adjective referring to **thoughts,** feelings or other information or processes of which the subject is not aware. As generally used, excludes material readily accessible to conscious awareness **(preconscious)** and thus designates processes or information not susceptible to **recall** at will. 2. Noun which designates the set of mental information or processes which are outside the reach of simple acts of recall and, more specifically in **psychoanalytic theory,** placed and maintained beyond recall by the mechanism of **repression.** Such information or processes are then regarded as the dynamic unconscious and constitute a part of the mind which indirectly influences conscious thoughts, attitudes and **behaviour.**

collective unconscious   *See* **Jung**.

undoing   An ego **defence mechanism** characterized by repetitive **behaviour** which symbolically prevents or reverses the consequences of some earlier unacceptable act. Commonly observed in **obsessional** disorders.

unipolar affective disorder   *See* **affective disorder.**

unreality feelings   *See* **depersonalization; derealization.**

unworthiness   Self-depreciation or negative evaluation of oneself and one's abilities, progressing to ideas or **delusions of unworthiness.** Common in primary **depressive** illness.

vaginismus   Spasm of the perivaginal muscles which occludes the vaginal opening and makes sexual intercourse difficult or impossible. The commonest cause of non-consummation of marriage, seemingly more so than that due to male impotence.

vandalism   Form of **delinquency,** consisting of destruction of property.

verbigeration   A verbal form of **stereotypy** in which, usually, meaningless words or sentences are repeatedly uttered, often in a recurrent and constant tone. Seen, for example, in **schizophrenic** patients who are institutionalized and socially uninvolved.

verstehende Psychologie   (Ger.) Interpretive **psychology;** a method of grasping the meanings and connections in the emotional life of a patient. **Jaspers** made important contributions to this field, which he contrasted with the different clinical approach of delimiting and describing the **symptoms, signs** and other aspects of a patient's experience. *See also* **phenomenology**.

visual agnosia   *See* **agnosia.**

volition   Voluntary activity consciously adopted by the individual, directed to a definite goal, and expressed in intention and decision. 2. The process of deciding upon a course of action without external pressure.

voodoo

voodoo Technically the name of a religion of the natives of Haiti. More generally used also to refer to West African, Brazilian, American negro and West Indian cults in which the **belief** that persons can be possessed by gods and spirits is axiomatic. The practice involves ridding or inducing **trance** and **possession** by **rituals** and **suggestion;** the effects can be very influential even causing **death** of individuals who are terrified by the forces presumed to be acting, in which they believe.

voyeurism Sexual deviation, consisting of repetitive looking at unsuspecting people, usually strangers, who are either naked, in the act of undressing, or engaging in sexual activity, as the repeatedly preferred or exclusive method of achieving sexual excitement.

wandering Moving about without purpose or direction. Sometimes used to mean out of one's **mind,** incoherent or rambling. In the sense of moving without purpose or direction, a common manifestation of childhood **conduct disorder** and of **organic** states in the elderly.

Watson, John Broadus (1878–1958) American psychologist, pioneer of **behaviourism**.

waxy flexibility *See* **flexibilitas cerea.**

Wechsler adult intelligence scale (WAIS) Multi-item **intelligence test** including both verbal and non-verbal material. The children's version is the Wechsler Intellingence Scale for Children (WISC).

Wernicke's syndrome **Delirium** in combination with squint due to paralysis of the eye muscles and an unsteady gait. Occurs in patients with **alcoholism** commonly and in conditions of persistent vomiting, due to a deficiency of vitamin B1 (thiamin).

Weyer, Johannes (1515–1588) The German physician, regarded by some as the first psychiatrist, whose book *Delusions of Witches* published in 1563 was a detailed exposé of the persecution of alleged **witches**.

Wilson's disease *See* **Hepatolenticular degeneration.**

witch A woman, rarely a man (warlock), who presumes to be able (or was presumed to be able) to use sorcery, usually for irreligious or wicked purposes.

working through

witchcraft The art of harnessing secret wisdom antagonistic to Christianity, and often involving sensuous sexual pleasures, **masochism, sadism** and allegiance to the Devil or Anti-Christ. The word is also used to describe less malignant studies of secret powers and unnatural rites, which most people feel to be totally bogus.

withdrawal Reduction of social contacts and assumption of a more introverted mode of existence. As a morbid process it may be a manifestation of numerous mental disorders.

alcohol withdrawal state Occurs when drinking is stopped by a person dependent on alcohol, or when the level of alcohol in the blood drops, leading to tension, shakiness of the hands, sweating, **insomnia** etc. An extreme is **delirium tremens.**

withdrawal state **Symptoms** occuring when the taking of a **drug** on which a person is dependent is interrupted.

withdrawal symptoms The appearance of **symptoms** following withdrawal of a **drug** on which a person is physically dependent. *See also* **addiction; dependence; tolerance.**

withdrawal syndrome Mental and physical disturbance consequent on cutting down or stopping intake of a psychopharmacologically active substance, e.g. alcohol, cocaine.

word association test A test invented by Galton in which a list of words is read to a subject who is asked to say the first word that comes into his mind in response. The test was mainly used by **Jung** in his studies of **psychosis** but has been little used in recent years for such clinical purposes. The technique remains of some interest as an investigatory tool in linguistics.

word salad A jumbled up sequence of spoken words and **neologisms** impossible to understand, which classically occurs in some chronic **schizophrenic** patients.

working through **Psychoanalytic** term; the process of time-consuming, repeated examination and **interpretation** of **neurotic** patterns until the associated and maladaptive **behaviour** has been understood and resolved. Usually used to describe the analytic work during a period when therapeutic progress seems arrested or slowed because of apparently intractable **resistance** on the part of the patient. Also, sometimes used to describe the process, outside the analytic situation, of psychic adjustment to a painful or difficult reality.

writer's cramp Disabling spasm of the small muscles of the hand caused by excessive muscle tone, which may be due to psychological tension or faulty writing habits.

Wundt, Wilhelm (1832–1920) German physiologist who was one of the founders of experimental **psychology**. He carried out studies of sensory **perception** and psychological associations, and developed a method of controlled introspection in the psychological laboratory. His major work *Grundzüge der physiologischen Psychologie*, published in 1873, laid the groundwork for psychology as a science.

X chromosome *See* **chromosomal sex**.

XO syndrome A **sex chromosome anomaly**, or monosomy. Though the commonest of the sex aneuploids to arise, 45X fetuses rarely survive until live birth. Development is along female lines but due to ovarian atrophy normal sexual development at **puberty** does not occur. Stature is small and various somatic anomalies arise, e.g. webbing of the neck. **Intelligence** is usually normal, though spatial aptitude may be impaired. Also known as Turner's syndrome or gonadal **dysgenesis**.

XXY karyotype Trisomy of the sex chromosomes resulting from non-disjunction at meiosis, occurring in 1 in 700 newborn males. Development is along normal male lines, except that the adult has small testes and is infertile. Less than average **intelligence**, late **puberty**, hypogonadism and gynaecomastia are common but not invariable. XXY males are typically taller than average *See also* **Klinfelter's syndrome, chromosomal sex; chromosome anomalies**.

XYY syndrome A **sex chromosome anomaly** occurring in 1 in 700 to 1000 live male births. Most affected individuals are free from obvious defects but tend to be taller than average and to have behavioural problems. Usually fertile, though tests show some abnormalities.

Zen (Zen Buddhism) Eastern teaching that a form of meditation which consists of contemplating one's essential nature, to the exclusion of all else, provides the way to true enlightenment. A transcendent and mystical approach to achieve enlightenment.

zygote The fertilized ovum.